T0127891

A NEW PARADIGM FOR INFORMED CONSENT

Irene S. Switankowsky

University Press of America,® Inc.
Lanham • New York • Oxford

Copyright © 1998 by
University Press of America,® Inc.
4720 Boston Way
Lanham, Maryland 20706

12 Hid's Copse Rd.
Cummor Hill, Oxford OX2 9JJ

Library of Congress Cataloging-in-Publication Data

Switankowsky, Irene S.
A new paradigm for informed consent / Irene S. Switankowsky.
p.   cm.
Includes bibliographical references and index.
l. Informed consent (Medical law). 2. Physician and patient. 3.
Autonomy (Psychology).   I. Title.
R724.S92   1998   610.69'6 —DC21   97-50149 CIP

ISBN 0-7618-1016-1 (cloth: alk. ppr.)

Contents

List of Figures and Tables

List of Figures   Page

List of Tables

Preface

This book has been developed with two goals in mind. First, I bring some of the key elements of informed consent into a unified theory that results in a new paradigm for informed consent based on an autonomy-enhancing model. To this end, I focus on some of the important aspects of informed consent and reinterpret them to fit the autonomy-enhancing model. Second, I redefine the physician-patient relationship in order to make sense of the relationship as an equal partnership between two individuals with the common goal of improving overall health and well-being. The view that the physician-patient relationship should be between equals is radical and controversial in comparison to the common view that a professional relationship sustains the relationship. However, if the view advocated in the book is acknowledged and practiced by the medical community, it will lessen the burdens of achieving an effective informed consent which is based on an autonomously derived decision by the patient in favour of a medical treatment.

Introduction

Informed consent has been (and still is) a complex and multi-faceted issue. There are two prevalent models for informed consent: (1) the traditional-harm-avoidance model which focuses on the physician as an authority in deciding which treatment the patient must undergo; and (2) the autonomy-enhancing model which insists that the patient must make an autonomous, reflective decision that is well informed in favor of a medical treatment. Physicians are typically reluctant to accept the autonomy-enhancing models of informed consent due to the psychological issues and complexities that may be involved. Physicians argue that these autonomy-enhancing models of informed consent are far too time consuming. Some may argue that to make the autonomy model a necessary condition for a patient to achieve an informed consent is to insist that the physician perform extra duties that are beyond their professional responsibilities. However, the irony is that most physicians are (at least minimally) cognizant that informed consent cannot be achieved without the patient's engaging in some sort of rational, autonomous decision making in favor of a treatment, when all the medical alternatives have been disclosed by the physician. Thus, mere "consent" does not constitute an "informed consent". No single signature on a form for any invasive medical procedure can be considered 'informed consent', though it may be a passive, unreflective form of 'consent' or acceptance.

Most of the medical procedures patients passively accept on the traditional harm-avoidance model (which is still prevalent today in many medical communities) are merely consented to. Isn't giving 'consent' similar in cognitive/psychological structure to giving an "informed consent"? One of the main themes of the book is the unequivocal repudiation of any possible analogue between 'mere consent' and 'informed consent'. All too often physicians tend to substitute 'consent' for 'informed consent'. I argue throughout the book that such a substitution is a grave error, and this for two reasons. *First*, the cognitive structure of the two experiential states is very different. Mere "consent" is passive, unreflective, non-autonomous, and is typically based on the physician's view of what is the best treatment for the patient. "Informed consent", on the other hand, involves an active, reflective, autonomous state of mind in which the patient makes a decision in favor of a medical treatment that is in the patient's perceived best interest. *Second*, when consent is viewed as equivalent to informed consent, the ultimate purpose of an informed consent is undermined. A substantially informed decision consists of an autonomous, reflective and rational decision by the patient in favor of a treatment which is well-understood and substantially disclosed by the physician, while mere "consent" consists of blind acceptance.

There is a vast amount of literature available on some of the key issues of informed consent, both from a theoretical and practical standpoint. If one compares ten paradigmatic texts on informed consent,[1] one finds that most of the texts only discuss one aspect of informed consent to the exclusion of any others. It is my contention that there are several essential conditions in order to effectively achieve a *substantially informed consent*. The key issues discussed in the texts that are essential for an informed consent to date are: autonomy, competency, promise keeping, truth telling, the principle of beneficence, and an effective physician-patient relationship. The union of these features of informed consent into a unified theory is a new view of informed consent, different from each of these theories since they left out something important that another theory did not recognize as being essential. These issues together form a complete account of informed consent, one that could be understood and emulated by all medical practitioners. Informed consent is much more complex than theorists originally believed it to be. The effectiveness and success of achieving an informed consent is determinate on the patient's personal idiosyncrasies which must be determined separately for each patient.

I argue that there are five conditions that could be formulated as a decision procedure for achieving an informed consent. The decision procedure for a 'substantially informed consent' is as follows:

Disclosure (D) + Understanding (U) + Rational Decision Making (RDM)
= Autonomous Decision
D + U + RDM +
Effective physician-Patient Relationship + Effective Communication
= Informed Consent

Thus, there are two stages in order to achieve a "substantially informed consent". First, the patient must achieve an autonomous decision through effective disclosure of the treatment alternatives available to him/her by the physician, must substantially understand the alternatives, and finally must rationally choose a treatment alternative that is in the patient's own best interest. Second, an effective physician-patient relationship and effective communication is necessary to achieve an autonomous decision and thus an informed consent. However, the first stage of informed consent is impossible to achieve without the second stage and, the first stage is impossible to achieve without a patient's capacity for autonomous and competent decisions, which are two foundational criteria for an informed consent. In the book, I devote one chapter to each of the two foundational criteria and the five conditions for informed consent. It has been my overall goal in the book to present the process of informed consent in detail, and to develop these conditions as decision procedures to ensure an informed consent is achieved. On the traditional, harm-avoidance model, the consent achieved is essentially a satisfaction of basic legal requirements, and thus cannot capture the complex processes involved in an informed consent. It then follows that the autonomy-enhancing model is the most realistic view to consider and accept since it ensures an informed consent. I will briefly outline the two foundational criteria and five conditions of a 'substantially' informed consent below for ease of comprehension.

I. Foundational Criteria for Informed Consent

(1) The foundational criteria of *autonomy* (examined in Chapter 1) insists that the patient must be capable of making substantially autonomous decisions to achieve an informed consent. The four aspects for determining whether a patient is autonomous are: (1) independence; (2) self-direction; (3) rationality/rational decision making; and (4) a genuine sense of self (i.e., what constitutes one's values, goals and life

plans). The last aspect is the most important for determining patient autonomy. An autonomous individual must have an accurate sense of his/her beliefs, values and goals, since important medical decisions must be made on the basis of such personal features of the self.

(2) The foundational criteria of *competency* (examined in Chapter 2) focuses on the mental ability of a patient to make a rational decision in favor of a medical treatment. Patient competency is difficult to define due to the lack of a precise definition in the legal and medical literature. I argue that there are three aspects of competency: (1) rational competence; (2) performance competence; and (3) reflective competence. Rational competence is an ability to make rational choices for oneself, choices that are consistent with one's beliefs, values, goals and life plans. Performance competence focuses on a patient's ability to make a rational choice in favor of a medical treatment by adequately understanding the nature of the treatment and the medical procedures. Reflective competence presupposes that the patient is able to not only understand all the information disclosed about the medical treatments and their risks and benefits, but also (if necessary) to re-evaluate his/her initial decision in favor of a certain treatment to determine whether it was rational.

II. Conditions for an Informed Consent

(1) *Disclosure of treatment alternatives* (examined in chapter 3). A physician, upon diagnosis of a patient's illness, must disclose all the treatment alternatives that are known by the physician and their risks and benefits. The patient and the physician must then eliminate the irrelevant alternatives together by determining which treatment(s) might be most appropriate for the patient given his/her values, goals, beliefs and medical condition. The process of elimination involves first removing all of the completely improbable medical treatment(s) and focusing more closely on the alternatives that are relevant and possible to administer. This process reduces information overload which is necessary for the patient to make a rational and autonomous decision in favor of a medical treatment.

There are two standards of disclosure: (1) the "professional standard" of disclosure, which is paternalistic in nature, and (2) the "reasonable person" standard of disclosure, which focuses on the patient as an autonomous person. The "reasonable person" standard of disclosure is the most promising for the autonomy-enhancing method of informed consent since it ensures that the patient is given all the necessary information to make a rational choice in favor of a medical treatment. The "reasonable person" standard of disclosure insists that the physician to disclose all the medical treatments that a reasonable, rational and reflective person would require to make a rational, well-informed and autonomous decision in favor of a treatment. The autonomy-enhancing model of informed consent is based on the "reasonable person" standard, since every patient must be considered competent to make his/her own decision based on the facts of medical treatments disclosed. The only time a patient should be deemed incompetent is if there is evidence that s(he) is not competent enough to make a rational and autonomous decision in favor of a treatment.

(2) *A substantial understanding of all the treatment alternatives* (examined in Chapter 4). On the autonomy-enhancing model, it is imperative for the patient to "substantially" understand all the relevant information that is disclosed to the physician about the medical treatments before the patient can make a rationally informed consent. A "substantial understanding" consists minimally of the physician's disclosing: (1) the risks and benefits of all the medical treatments available, (2) the pain and hardship that may have to be endured with each treatment alternative, (3) the recuperation time for each treatment alternative, (4) the diagnostic methodology for each treatment, and (5) an overall assessment of the relevant medical treatments to determine which is most beneficial for the particular patient given his/her medical situation.

This process ensures that the patient will make a reflective and autonomous choice about a medical treatment, one that is consistent with his/her values, goals, beliefs and life plans. The patient should make a decision in favor of a medical treatment that is consistent with his/her own experiences as an autonomous person whose life will necessarily be affected by certain treatment alternatives. Thus, on the autonomy-enhancing model, the five features of understanding outlined above are necessary conditions for achieving an informed decision that is substantially understood in favor of a treatment alternative.

(3) *Rational Decision Making* (examined in Chapter 5). On the autonomy-enhancing model, a patient must make a substantially rational decision for an informed consent to be achieved. A "substantially rational" decision is: (i) free from biases and inappropriate heuristics, and (ii) based on a substantially reflective awareness to avoid any errors in initial judgment.

(i) *Biases and Heuristics.* In order for a patient's decision to be rational, it must not rely on extraneous factors which are strictly irrelevant to the decision. For instance, a patient may initially frame a medical treatment solely on the basis of some remotely possible risks, say of dying, while avoiding any of the important benefits, say of short term pain for long term gain. This may be due to a previous negative experience in the patient's life, such as his/her father passing away while undergoing a similar treatment. Thus, the patient may use that painful memory as an erroneous justification for not undergoing the medical treatment. Such a decision isn't rational since the patient failed to rationally assess all the medical treatment but "framed" the treatment using the biases of past experiences. The risk of dying as a result of the treatment became a bias through which the patient irrationally 'framed' the treatment. If the patient fails to be reflective about his/her initial decision, the patient's decision would be irrational and thus non-autonomous, since the patient's decision was swayed by emotions that were not strictly relevant to the particular treatment that the patient was to undergo. One way to avoid such irrational decisions is for the patient to "step-back" from his/her original decision and reassess the decision.

(ii) *Substantial Reflective Awareness.* Reflective awareness is a second-order operation on the initial decision process, a way of reassessing an original decision. This is a method of "stepping-back" from our initial judgments, and reinterpreting the information disclosed and our assessment of the information. If a biased decision is made in favor of a medical treatment (as would be the case if the patient decided against a treatment option due to a prior death in the family), the patient would have to reflect a second time on the benefits and risks of the treatment, and hopefully come to realize that his/her initial decision was biased and thus irrational. A reassessment that is based on a second-order reflection by the patient of the treatment risks and benefits could eventually lead to a rational decision about the treatment. Reflection is crucial in bringing about an autonomous decision about a treatment alternative.

xiv

(4) *An Effective physician-Patient Relationship* (examined in Chapter 6). On the autonomy-enhancing model, the physician-patient relationship is characterized as a partnership based on mutual trust and respect, in which the two individuals must be treated as moral equals. An effective physician-patient relationship is one in which the two individuals relate to each other in a cordial and caring manner. The physician must know his/her patient's personal idiosyncrasies such as his/her values, goals, beliefs and life plans, whereas the patient should know the physician's professional idiosyncrasies such as his/her medical expertise or gaps in medical knowledge. Such personal information can help the physician and patient interact with each other more readily. There are benefits to having such personal knowledge about a patient, one of which is the ability to assess whether a patient's medical decision in favor of a treatment is out of character.

This may be especially pertinent for a patient who feels vulnerable due to the uncertainties of the medical context. Compatible physician-patient relationships are especially desirable since the process of informed consent is thereby facilitated and an autonomous, rational and reflective decision will therefore be more readily achieved. Compatibility between physician and patient also has an effect on a patient's overall process of recuperation after treatment. When a patient feels genuinely cared for, it can have a considerably positive influence on the patient's recovery due to the encouragement and confidence that is developed by the physician. The patient will feel much more confident and s(he) will have a much more positive attitude towards life and his/her diagnosis and treatment. No such benefits are possible on the traditional, paternalistic, harm-avoidance model.

(5) *Effective Communication between Patient and Physician* (examined in Chapter 7). All significant human relationships are developed through open, honest communication between the two individuals, and this is also the case with the physician and patient relationship. Effective communication between physician and patient consists of honesty, promise-keeping in the form of confidentiality, and a sympathetic attitude between the patient and physician. Each of these features of communication strengthen the effectiveness of the physician-patient relationship and brings it to a level where the patient and physician can feel confident about their relationship in a context that is prone to various vulnerabilities due to a patient's illness and a physician's medical uncertainties.

Effective communication is therefore a necessary condition for achieving an effective physician-patient relationship. A foundational element of effective communication is honesty. Honesty may be characterized as an open and forthright disclosure by the physician of the medical alternatives that are available to the patient. This is essential for a patient to make a rational, reflective and substantially understood decision in favor of a particular treatment. When a physician and patient are honest with one another, they hold certain personal information that is shared between them concealed from all third parties (be it relatives or medical staff). The patient, in turn, must be honest by asking the physician further questions about a medical alternative(s) if s(he) has not understood some aspect of it. The physician must trust that the patient has given a substantially informed consent, and also have a sympathetic attitude toward his/her patient in order to feel what it would be like to experience a similar medical ailment. All these features of honesty help to nurture an effective physician-patient relationship.

I propose a new paradigm for informed consent (examined in chapter 8) based on autonomous, reflective, rational, substantially understood medical treatments that are substantially disclosed to the patient. The autonomy-enhancing model developed throughout the book is distinctive since it ensures that a new and promising ideology of informed consent is impossible to develop by strongly holding onto the traditional, harm-avoidance model (which is presently prevalent in medical communities). When physicians recognize this, a paradigm shift from the traditional, harm-avoidance model to the autonomy-enhancing model will occur. If this book is successful, it will help physicians recognize the importance of ensuring that their patients have given an informed consent rather than mere consent. This will create a paradigm shift in medicine that is necessary to improve the quality of patient care, and to ensure that an informed consent is given. Nothing less could count as an 'informed consent'.

III. How to Read the Book

The book will be most effective if it is read consecutively from chapter to chapter since each chapter presupposes the knowledge of the previous chapter in order to ensure proper understanding. The first two chapters may be the most difficult to understand due to the vagueness associated with notions of autonomy and competency as it relates to the medical situation. The first chapter on autonomy is difficult because it attempts to define a philosophical concept that is riddled with psychological complexities and individual particularities. It is recommended that the first chapter be read and then perhaps re-read to facilitate understanding. Chapter two is also difficult since it focuses on the controversial notion of determining patient competency, which is a multi-faceted and complicated endeavor to achieve. This chapter should also perhaps be read carefully. The remaining chapters in the book should not pose too many problems to the medical community and to any general readers.

IV. The Intended Audience for the Book

This book was primarily written for medical professionals and especially medical doctors who must ensure daily that an informed consent is given for routine and invasive medical procedures. The book is also written for laypersons who are interested in being more informed about how they can ensure that they give an informed consent in favor of a medical procedure. This book is not intended as a philosophical treatise on the theoretical aspects of informed consent; instead, I have approached the topic mostly from a practical perspective. In other words, I discuss informed consent from within the trenches of the medical situation divorced from its theoretical ramifications which cannot really touch some of the inherent complexities that physicians and patients experience daily.

Notes

1. The ten texts on informed consent are as follows:

   1. T. Beauchamp, & J. Childress, *Principles of Biomedical Ethics.* (New York: Oxford University Press, 1979.
   2. Ruth Faden & Tom Beauchamp, *A History and Theory of Informed Consent.* (New York: Oxford University Press, 1986).
   3. Jay Katz. *The Silent World of physician and Patient.* (New York: Free Press, 1984).
   4. Stephen Lammers, & Allen Verhey. *On Moral Medicine.* (Oxford: Oxford University Press, 1985).
   5. Thomas, John, E., & Waluchow, Wilfred. *Well and Good: Case Studies in Biomedical Ethics.* (Ontario: Broadview Press, Ltd., 1987).
   6. Donald Van De Veer. *Paternalistic Intervention: The Moral Bounds of Benevolence.* (New Jersey: Princeton University Press, 1986).
   7. Robert M, Veatch. *A Theory of Medical Ethics.* (New York: Basic Books, Inc., 1981).
   8. Richard Warner. *Morality in Medicine.* (Sherman Oaks: Alfred, 1980).
   9. Richard Wright. *Human Values in Health Care: The Practice of Ethics.* (New York: McGraw Hill, 1988).
   10. Peter Young. *Personal Autonomy: Beyond Negative and Positive Liberty.* (London: Croom Helm, 1986).

Chapter 1

Autonomy as the Foundation
of Informed Consent

This chapter outlines a theory of autonomy that is essential for determining whether a patient's decision in favor of a medical treatment is based on properly informed consent. Autonomy is the foundation of properly informed consent since in the absence of an autonomous decision, informed consent becomes mere consent. Consents are not properly informed unless they are autonomously decided upon by the patient. Autonomy is a complex cognitive-relational state of affairs that varies in degree and quality between individuals. The more morally developed, reflective, and educationally informed an individual is, the more autonomous will his/her decisions be. Autonomy, or freely choosing, ranges from minimal to adequate or strongly adequate depending on the individual and the particular (medical) situation. Medical vulnerabilities, severe pain, and anxiety could also decrease a person's autonomy either due to the uncertainties that are implicit in certain medical treatments or the prognosis of the patient's illness.

I. Harm-avoidance vs. Autonomy enhancing model of informed consent

There are two paradigms of consent that are prevalent in the medical context:

(1)   the harm avoidance model of informed consent; and
(2)   the autonomy-enhancing model of informed consent.

(1) *The harm avoidance paradigm* of informed consent is the common, even standard framework within which physicians operate. Due to the rapidly increasing technology in medicine and the development of dangerous or high-risk surgery, physicians agree that they must obtain consent from a patient, disclosing the risks of the treatment involved, and that the patient must give an informed consent on the basis at least of his/her minimal understanding of these risks. The thesis of this book is that the minimalist disclosure that is implicit in the framework of the harm avoidance paradigm of informed consent is insufficient for preserving a patient's autonomy and cannot ensure that the patient's decision is autonomous. Thus, on the harm avoidance model, consent to treatment is usually considered to be a mere legal formality of signing a consent form. This formality does not honor and respect a patient's individual and personal autonomy, which is the ultimate purpose of obtaining an informed consent.

According to the harm avoidance model, most of the intricate facets of the treatment and even some of the remote risks with the various medical treatments need not be revealed to the patient. In contrast, on the autonomy-enhancing model, *all* the details and medical treatments must be disclosed and discussed in detail with the patient; in addition, all the risks and benefits of each medical treatment must be disclosed, and not only the medical treatments chosen by the physician. The patient's responses may sometimes be influenced by the physician's presentation of the facts of the treatment. The ultimate purpose of informed consent is to ensure that the patient makes an autonomous, rational, reflective, well-understood decision about a medical procedure or treatment alternative that s(he) believes will be most beneficial. In short, the ultimate purpose of properly informed consent is to protect a patient's autonomy under all medical circumstances.

Informed consent is necessary because of the possible infringement of autonomy due to certain medical treatments and their effect on the patient. Infringement of autonomy is a serious moral issue that must not be overlooked by physicians. On the autonomy-enhancing theory of informed consent developed in the book, the primary purpose for informed consent is to respect a patient's autonomy even if this overrides the duty a medical professional has of eliminating as much anxiety as possible about a medical treatment. Another way of putting the same point is that the physician must respect the patient as a person and a moral agent before s(he) can protect the patient from harm.

II. Definition of Autonomy[1]

There is a multitude of definitions of autonomy in the literature, many of which are formally similar, yet distinct in certain idiosyncratic ways. (Beauchamp and Childress, 1979, 56-57) offer one general definition of autonomy that is a good starting point:

> Autonomy is a form of personal liberty of action where the individual determines his or her own course of action in accordance with a plan chosen by himself or herself. The autonomous person is one who not only deliberates about and chooses such plans but who is capable of acting on the basis of such deliberations, just as a truly independent government has autonomous control of it territories and policies.

From this definition, we can identify several general features of the concept of autonomy: (1) self-government in the sense of being master of oneself in actions and inner being; (2) reflectiveness about one's actions and inner states of affairs; (3) a solid, clearly known set of life plans and goals that cohere with one's actions and behaviors; (4) overall control of one's actions and behaviors leading to fulfillment and a wholeness of being; and (5) a fully developed sense of person -- a sense of who one is.

If the ideal were that of *complete* or *total* autonomy, and every patient would have to make completely autonomous decisions in favor of a medical treatment in order to achieve informed consent. However, very few of us are completely autonomous. What is required, in contrast, is that complete autonomy should be thought of as an ideal that each individual should strive to achieve, but that the achievement will come in gradations and degrees. What would be beneficial is a set of heuristics for determining whether we are more or less autonomous to make a rational decision. Our sense of autonomy will be weakened or strengthened, depending on the medical situation. We cannot be expected to exercise the same degree of autonomy in each situation. This is especially the case in medical situations where patients may feel threatened or vulnerable due to illness, continuous pain, or having taken certain medications that may cause their sense of autonomy to be diminished.

When illness sets in (especially chronic illness),[2] an individual's existence takes on a different quality because illness is a lived experience. The alleviation of pain and suffering is foremost on the patient's mind, and his/her overall coherence of life plans and goals may become distorted. What often comes to the surface when a patient becomes ill are his/her basic personality traits and values that are important to his/her overall sense of inner being. Character traits such as kindness, altruism, pleasantness and honesty, and unkindness, or egoism, unpleasantness and irritability (depending on the particular person's personality) come to the foreground. A careful observation of these basic features of personality, will assist a medical practitioner in determining what is important to a patient, and assist him/her in understanding what medical information to disclose to a particular patient in achieving an informed consent.

No two individuals will likely have the same sense of autonomy since it differs in degree and kind. Some have a more developed sense of autonomy than others. There are some conditional heuristics[3] that could be used by physicians to determine the degree or intensity of a patient's quality of autonomy. This is a difficult question to answer. Perhaps a general rule of thumb for determining a patient's sense of autonomy is the degree of self-knowledge and reflectiveness that a patient demonstrates. This may implicitly show that the patient has a more developed sense of autonomy than a patient who acts on the whims and immediate responses of the moment. However, a person could be reflective and still not be autonomous, if some of the other features of autonomy listed above are absent.

III. Two Principles of Autonomy

There are two fundamental principles of all autonomous choice, decision and action: (1) respect for persons; and (2) self-rule or self-determination.5

(1) *The Respect for Persons.*[4] A physician must respect the patient's unique and distinctly individual values, commitments and character traits. When a physician displays such respect by seeking to understand the intricacies of the patient, the physician respects the patient as a person. The physician must determine the patient's goals and values prior to disclosing the detailed medical information about the medical treatments. In this way, the physician will avoid communicating medical information that may be generally relevant but not specifically pertinent to the patient.

Let us consider the following case as an illustration of how the physician must respect his/her patient:

A patient (Helen) is diagnosed with a cancerous growth on her ankle, and she must have it removed. There is a further risk that the patient will have her leg amputated at a later date. Should the physician disclose the latter risk to the patient, even if it may be a remote possibility?

Consider that the physician has the following information about the patient under consideration:

(i) the patient is an athlete and would like to join the Olympic games to compete in the finals within a year;

(ii) the patient is an honest and disciplined person who values doing the best she can be at all times;

(iii) the patient is also a well known and prolific philosopher who is devoted to academic pursuits;

(iv) the patient is rational and has a well developed life plan, values and beliefs, forming a coherent set of beliefs that s(he) is able to commit her life to; and

(v) the patient is easy to communicate with due to the knowledge and clarity of her intrinsic values and extrinsic life plans.

If the physician is honest--which s(he) must be otherwise the patient's autonomy and sense of personhood will be violated--s(he) should disclose the risk of amputation to the patient. Since one of the patient's known goals is to run in the finals of the Olympics, the amputation would render such a goal impossible. Since the patient is a rational decision maker, she will probably choose to undergo the treatment and to accept the inevitable possibility of having her leg amputated, but also accept the impossibility of competing in the Olympics which will subsequently become a subsidiary goal of her life. The patient's life may turn out to be less fulfilling since one of her important goals in life (i.e., to compete in the Olympics) will have come to an abrupt end; however, it would not lack everything that is valuable to her since she still has a philosophical career. Thus, detailed information about a patient is critical to make autonomous decisions about his/her medical treatment(s) and well-being.

On the autonomy-enhancing model of informed consent, the physician must disclose all the information of the treatment and all the risks involved. Even if the physician was only aware that the patient was a philosopher and not an athlete (or vice versa), s(he) should disclose the medical information about the risk of amputation. Such complete disclosure may be criticized by some as being far too stringent as a criteria of autonomy; however, the model should be used if only as a guideline for achieving a properly informed consent. Respecting a patient's autonomy is a primary reason for informed consent, and the autonomy that is preserved must be of the highest quality. The harm-avoidance model of consent fails since it doesn't focus on the person as a rational agent but on a sick body. Persons and their lives are affected by their illness, since illness is a lived experience, and is not something that can be abstracted from the person as a whole. This will be the dominant theme of the chapters that follow since it is one of the key justifications of the autonomy-enhancing model for informed consent.

(2) *Self-rule or self-determination*[5] is the individual's ability to legislate rules for oneself and to govern his/her behavior according to his/her own plans, goals and values of the person. A person that is self-directed usually knows what is in his/her best interest, and his/her life displays and executes unified and coherent life plans. Such a person

would know the parameters of his/her tolerance for pain; his/her ability to cope with pain; the infringement that pain imposes on his/her concentration, memory, and reflective capabilities; and the degree to which his/her autonomy is hampered when s(he) is ill. If the patient communicates such facts as clearly as possible to the physician, s(he) will be in a better position to ensure that the patient makes an autonomous decision about treatment.

The foundational feature of autonomy consists of a coherent set of values, goals, beliefs and life plans that weave a distinct individual into a coherent whole. An adequate sense of autonomy is based on a developed set of beliefs that endure over time and which governs the individual's behavior in expressing consistent values and goals used to make important decisions about one's life, as is the case when a patient makes a decision about a particular medical treatment. Each of a person's beliefs ideally should reinforce his/her unique values, beliefs and goals. Every individual must act on the basis of these foundational beliefs and values, and any situation that threatens the unity of these values and beliefs is to be avoided.

It must again be stressed that this sense of autonomy is an ideal and perhaps not realistic for some. However, the closer an individual can approach this ideal, the more consistent will the patient's decisions be to his/her deeply held beliefs, goals and values, and thus the more autonomous will his/her decisions be in favor of a medical treatment. This is especially the case when making a properly informed consent. For instance, some courageous patients may chose a treatment that a less courageous patient wouldn't even think of as an option. A patient that can endure severe pain would perhaps refrain from taking certain medications while another patient that is more sensitive to pain would gladly accept the medication and tolerate the side effects to relieve his/her discomfort.

Autonomy varies from patient to patient, and this may make it difficult for health professionals to know how well developed their patient's sense of autonomy is prior to making a decision in favor of a medical treatment. A time consuming, but nonetheless effective way that physicians could determine his/her patient's sense of autonomy is to have extended informal conversations with the patient. In the process, the physician will be able to determine important personal facts about the patient's beliefs, values and goals that will give him/her a sense of whether the patient's sense of autonomy is mature, immature or moderately developed. As already mentioned, the more mature a patient's autonomy, the more informed will be his/her decision for a given medical treatment. Determining the range of a patient's autonomy is critical to ensuring that a patient gives an informed consent, since autonomy is the foundation of informed consent.

IV. Negative, Positive and Moderate Views of Autonomy

There are two extreme views of autonomy. The extreme *negative view of autonomy* holds that most individuals are, in principle, incapable of making autonomous decisions, and the notion that they have autonomy is a myth. The extreme *positive view* of autonomy holds that individuals are fully autonomous beings with respect to every action and decision. There is also a *moderate view of autonomy* which holds that autonomy comes in degrees. This is the view I will adopt in the book.

On *the extreme negative view*, it is held that most individuals are in principle incapable of making autonomous decisions since no individual can have a completely coherent set of values, life goals and beliefs. In effect, such individuals have an inconsistent set of beliefs and goals. In addition, on this view, most individuals are irrational decision makers because they can never know what is in their best interest, and therefore can never make fully autonomous decisions. Individuals do not have any real freedom to choose because they choose one thing and then typically do something contradictory. Such individuals fail to have an adequate knowledge of themselves, owing to an incoherent set of beliefs, and an inability to effectively correct the incoherence. Their decisions will tend to be based merely on the incidental features of the particular situation at hand, and the emotions they feel at the moment. Their decision will therefore not be autonomous.

On the moderate view promoted here, it is admitted that there are such persons and that they can be easily persuaded or even "voluntarily" coerced into accepting decisions in favor of a medical treatment they should not accept if they were able to reflect on them autonomously. Such individuals will need the help of professional psychotherapists and other medical professionals to achieve a properly informed consent. They are typically influenced by biases, prejudices, and heuristics that are irrelevant to their decision. It is denied, however, that there is a multitude of such persons -- certainly they do not make up the bulk of humanity. The moderate view holds that capacities for autonomous decision appears as a range, or scale, from the very minimal to the maximal capacity. If such inconsistencies became noticeable, the patient is probably lacking in reflective skills and capabilities that make him/her a rational decision maker and therefore an autonomous individual. It is perhaps controversial to assert that autonomy is based on a skill that may be developed by individuals. It is not, however, controversial to assert that autonomy is a disposition that is capable of development through learning. Individuals can become progressively more reflective about their values, goals, beliefs and life plans, and thus can become more autonomous through practice. The more one engages in reflection, the more reflective one becomes. Physicians must try to patiently engage in effective communication with such patients in order to bring about an attitude of reflectiveness that ensures that the patient's decision be minimally autonomous. If time is an issue, trained medical assistants, psychologists, or nurses could help in the initial processes of this intricate and complex examination.

On *the extreme positive view*, it is held that most individuals have a mature and well-developed sense of autonomy. Such individuals are fully aware of all their values, goals and life plans, and have developed a coherent set of beliefs such that they are capable of complete rational decisions.[6] Such individuals would always make only those rational decisions that are consistent with their overall values and goals. For instance, in medical situations, such individuals would know exactly how sensitive they are and how much pain they can and will endure. Physicians always have a hope of treating fully rational and autonomous patients; however, this rarely ever happens. Usually physicians must help patients to achieve rational decisions through detailed discussion and investigation. If every individual was fully autonomous in this sense, properly informed consent would not be a problem to achieve. However, this is far from the case.

The Moderate View holds that most individuals have, for the most part, an adequately developed sense of autonomy. This view presumes that some individuals have a partially coherent set of beliefs, goals and aspirations; i.e., that at least some of his/her values and goals cohere with their overall set of beliefs, and these beliefs form life plans that are consistent for the most part. However, this coherence does not apply to all of a patient's values and beliefs. Some of the patient's beliefs may be incoherent and in need of amendment. Such individuals are usually reflective about their decisions, especially those decisions that will substantially affect their well being, as is the case in medical situations. It is still possible, of course, for such individuals to make irrational decisions, but the likelihood that s(he) will do so is not as great, given proper advising by the physician. Such individuals typically have an adequate set of coherent beliefs that weave his/her sense of personhood, with some inconsistencies around the periphery.

Typically, advocates of the autonomy-enhancing model argue for the stronger view of autonomy (Faden and Beauchamp, 1986). They argue that patients must be "substantially" autonomous to give an informed consent, and on the autonomy-enhancing model of informed consent this may, on the surface, seem to be necessary. I disagree with this contention primarily because it is too unrealistic; most patients would fail the test miserably, making properly informed consent impossible to achieve. Thus, on the view I propose, "moderately autonomous" decisions could also lead to a properly informed consent. Most individuals only have a moderate recognition of their values, goals and life plans, and hardly any individuals have a completely coherent set of such beliefs and values.

Achieving an informed consent for such an individual may be difficult but not unachievable. A process of effective communication between physician and patient is a necessary condition for informed consent. The patient may learn a lot about him/herself through this process, and the physician will become aware of his/her patient's decision making capabilities. The physician will then be able to decide whether his/her patient has given a properly informed consent that is autonomous and based on his/her deeply held beliefs. Most reflective individuals fit into this category of autonomy and most individuals could be characterized as having an adequate or moderate sense of autonomy. We all know some aspects or features about ourselves that are coherent, whereas other features of our personhood and values are unknown.

V. Determining Patient Autonomy

There are four ways that a physician could evaluate patient autonomy. These are:

(1) independence;
(2) self-direction;
(3) rationality or rational decision making; and
(4) a developed sense of self.

(1) *Independence*. The physician must assess whether the patient acts on the basis of his/her own reasoned decisions, or whether the patient depends on others for his/her decisions. There is an important distinction between asking for suggestions from others, and then making our own decision, in contrast to being dependent on others to make decisions on our behalf. The difference is subtle but the physician should be able to determine a patient's independence by asking him/her some questions about treatment and observing how s(he) makes decisions.[7]

(2) *Self-Direction*. Self-direction is related to independence, although it has a distinct meaning and significance. Self-direction can be assessed by the physician by observing a patient's capacity for deliberation, which consists of the thinking processes that an individual undergoes in making decisions. A patient may be independent, yet not have adequate self-directive skills. Ideally, a patient's deliberative skills must mirror his/her values, goals, and life plans. Certain medical treatments will be completely unsatisfactory to the patient, whereas others may be tolerable and satisfactory. The decisions about these treatments are self-directed to the extent that a patient could assess his/her medical treatments by consulting his/her inner beliefs, values, life goals and personal character traits. Self-direction in itself has little to do with rationality, and more to do with individual initiative in deliberating on the personal features of an individual's physical and psychological make-up.

(3) *Rationality or Rational Decision Making.*   Given a patient's particular idiosyncrasies, it is possible for a physician to determine whether the patient's decision for treatment is rational by observing his/her thinking processes. The physician must determine the patient's medical history and psychological/personal information prior to assessing whether his/her patient is capable of making a rational decision. This is most successfully achieved when the physician engages in effective communication with the patient over a period of time, and comes to an intuitive evaluation and assessment of his/her general responses and attitudes. Over time, a physician may develop a set of criteria that s(he) could use to determine whether a particular patient's decision in favor of a medical treatment is likely to be rational. There is no one single objective, universal characterization of rationality that applies to each and every patient without exception. Instead, each patient will have a slightly different set of criteria for rationality; thus, the criteria are subjective and must be determined for each patient separately.

There are two senses of rationality in decision making:

(i) The *formal sense of rationality* refers to consistency and to the defects in the structure of a patient's deliberations, such as self-contradictions, inconsistencies, fallacious thinking processes and so on. If such defects are consistently involved in a patient's deliberations, his/her decision will be irrational.
(ii) The *material sense of rationality* involves the beliefs, values and commitments that form the content of the decision. Again, if the beliefs and values of a patient are consistently inconsistent, it can be assumed that the patient cannot make autonomous decisions about his/her treatments that will satisfy the general requirements of rationality which focuses heavily on consistency.

Thus, both the structure and content of a patient's deliberations must be taken into consideration for a decision to be rational (i.e., consistent) and to satisfy the criteria for an autonomous decision about a particular treatment.

(4) *A Developed Sense of Self.* The self is the inner core of an individual, the dispositions that reinforce his/her goals, values, beliefs, likes and dislikes and so on. The self influences decisions, and especially medical decisions for treatment since the patient is usually deeply affected by medical diseases, procedures and medications. The patient must decide for him/herself precisely what s(he) will endure based on his/her inner self. The inner self is not hidden or mysterious but something we can each become aware of through introspection and by observing our actions and responses over time. The physician can understand his/her patient by observing his/her behavior and determining whether s(he) has a mature, well-developed sense of self and self knowledge that is reliable, or whether s(he) has an inconsistent, irrational sense of self that may result in irrational decisions.

Much more will be said about rational decision making in Chapter 5. For the present, however, I will outline the conditions that the physician can use as guidelines for predicting or determining a patient's autonomy. It is sometimes difficult to accurately assess how developed a patient's sense of autonomy really is; nevertheless, unless a physician achieves this, s(he) may inadequately assess whether the patient has the capacity for giving an autonomous decision and thus an informed consent. The ultimate purpose of informed consent is to ensure that the patient could make an autonomous decision that is consistent with his/her goals, values and life plans.

Notes

1. I am assuming that every person is in principle capable of autonomous decision and action. The harm avoidance model, while it necessarily assumes this capacity, does not necessarily require the exercise of the capacity.
2. "Chronic illness" consists of a long term disease which causes severe pain and discomfort such as certain cancers, AIDS, and multiple sclerosis, just to name a few. There is no short term medical treatments for such diseases; instead, the patient must become adapted to the pain and discomfort which becomes a part of his/her life.

"Acute illness" in contrast is a short term medical disability that is usually cured by medication and/or surgery. Patients only endure pain and discomfort for a short term, and then such patients become healthy.

3. The "conditional heuristics" consist of the five conditions that are necessary for achieving an informed consent. These are: (1) disclosure (examined in chapter 3); (2) understanding (examined in chapter 4); (3) rational decision making (examined in chapter 5); (4) effective physician-patient relationship (examined in chapter 6); and (5) effective communication (examined in chapter 7). These five conditions form a set of conditions for a decision procedure to achieve an informed consent.

4. There are two ways of characterizing the principle of autonomy: (1) an agency-type account of autonomy, which focuses on the features of personhood (i.e., beliefs, values, and life plans) that are crucial to determining whether a person is autonomous; and (2) a consequentialist account of autonomy, where the consequences of an individual's actions are of foremost importance in determining whether one's actions are autonomous. The two principles of autonomy that I referred to above are Kantian in origin. However, they are not identical with Kant's *Groundwork of the Metaphysics of Morals* since I avoid universalizing the two principles of autonomy.

5. However, I do rely on two Kantian principles. The first is the principle of respect for persons. Kant writes:

"Now I say that man, and in general every rational being, exists as an end in himself and not merely as a means to be arbitrarily used by this or that will. He must in all his actions, whether directed to himself or to other rational beings, always be regarded at the same time as an end." *Groundwork of the Metaphysics of Morals* (p.34).

The respect that is implied in this passage is a feeling of awe towards another individual. I argue that the patient and physician must have a similar regard for one another, without some of the emotional connotations that awe may invite. Kant only aimed at an intellectual awe for a person's unique character traits and moral laws, and this is also my aim here.

6. The second is the principle of self-rule. Kant writes:

"A rational being must always regard himself as legislator in a kingdom of ends rendered possible by freedom of the will, whether as member or as sovereign." *Groundwork of the Metaphysics of Morals* (p.40) .

Self-rule implies that an individual can make decisions that are based on his/her own beliefs, values, goals and life plans. My account of autonomy is therefore non-consequentialist in principle since the two principles of autonomy are based more on agency and personhood than on the consequences for actions. Consequentialism is the view that the rightness or wrongness, and/or goodness or badness of an action is solely dependent on the results the action produces.
7. This is the view advocated by Ruth R. Faden and Tom L. Beauchamp. *A History and Theory of Informed Consent* (New York: Oxford University Press,1986), "The Concept of Autonomy", Chapter 7, p.238-240. They argue for a theory of 'substantial autonomy' as a necessary condition for achieving an informed consent that is 'fully understood' and 'completely uncontrolled'. This is an unrealistic picture on the account of informed consent that is advocated throughout the book.
8. J. Chrisley Hackler, "Patient Autonomy in Medicine", in David H. Smith's *Respect and Care in Medical Ethics* (Lanham, MD: University Press of America, 1984).

Chapter 2

Patient Competency

Assessing patient competence is perhaps one of the most difficult aspects of informed consent, since there is little agreement as to the exact boundaries of mental competence. The legal definition of incompetence in the United States is too broad and vague to be helpful in medical situations; incompetence is "that mental condition which renders him incapable of taking care of his person or handling and managing his estate".[1] This, of course, is the most extreme type of incompetence, dealing with patients in a coma or in a comatose state. On this legal definition, unless a patient is incompetent in this extreme sense, s(he) still has the ability to make a properly informed consent about a medical intervention. This legal definition of competence is too narrow since almost anyone, except a patient that has significant mental defects, is competent enough to manage his/her estate to some degree and therefore is capable of making medical decisions. Thus, the legal definition fails to give sufficient emphasis to the patient making an autonomous decision, the physician's disclosure of the medical treatments, and a patient's understanding of the treatments.

I. Characterization of Patient Competency

The competence required for informed consent on the autonomy-enhancing model is complex and multi-faceted since it involves a significant amount of rational perspicuity. In order to assess whether a patient is competent, the physician must have an adequate knowledge of the patient's personal, psychological and medical history in order to determine whether s(he) is competent. Competence is not an all or nothing notion, as the legal definition suggests. There are two extremes of competence, both of which are misguided, since most patients fall somewhere between the two extremes. On the one hand, there is the type of incompetent patient who is severely mentally handicapped, or the patient in a coma. In this case, some form of paternalism or surrogate consent is necessary, and informed consent takes the form of mere consent by a third party. On the other hand, there is the completely competent patient who knows every aspect of his/her life plans, goals and values and has communicated them adequately to the physician so that s(he) is convinced that his/her patient knows about all the treatments and has autonomously chosen among them.

This chapter will focus on the notion of competence between these two extremes since at either the severely incompetent or completely competent stages, lack of competence or complete competence is readily determined without much difficulty. For instance, in the case of the severely incompetent, it is apparent that an informed consent cannot be achieved by the patient him/herself since his/her decision will inevitably be nonautonomous (this is represented in the 0-20% competency rate in Figure 2.1). Further, for the fully competent patient, there is no difficulty to achieve an informed consent since with complete self-knowledge and self-understanding the patient ensures that whatever decision is made it will cohere with his/her overall beliefs, values and life goals (this is represented in the 0-100 range in Figure 2.1). The most difficult cases of competence for informed consent lie somewhere between the fully competent and fully incompetent. There is a wide range of qualities of competence that ranges from poor to adequate to substantial (see Figure 2.1). The range of competence typically depends on a patient's educational background, intelligence, beliefs, values, ethical outlook, decision making skills, reflective ability, and rationality. All of these factors enter into patient competence, and the physician must use these factors as guidelines to assess a patient's competence.

II. The Three Parameters of Competency

Three parameters of competence[2] are essential to the autonomy-enhancing model:

(1) rational competence;
(2) performance competence; and
(3) reflective competence.

Rational competence and reflective competence are closely related and, although discussed separately, in some respects they reinforce one other. Rational competence is the ability to form a reasonable decision, one that is consistent and compatible with one's beliefs, values, and long/short term goals. Reflective competence requires rational competence in that the latter is minimally necessary for the former. Reflective competence is the ability to be self-consciously aware of one's personal values and goals simultaneously. This is especially an important issue for informed consent since in order for the patient to make a rational decision in favor of a medical treatment, the patient must reflect on his/her deeply held values and beliefs.

These three parameters of competence are objective requirements for an informed consent since they are empirical features for determining whether a patient is capable of providing an informed consent. In subsequent chapters, I outline the subjective conditions for informed consent that depend on a physician's knowledge of the patient's personal values, goals, beliefs, and life plans. The subjective requirements include: physician disclosure of medical treatments, understanding between physician and patient, rational decision making, developing an effective patient-physician relationship, and effective communication. At the initial stage of assessment the physician must decide whether a patient is minimally competent to give an informed consent. The objective criteria constitutes the minimal conditions for informed consent, while the subjective features are maximal conditions. On the autonomy-enhancing model of informed consent, both the objective criteria and subjective conditions are essential if there is to be an informed consent.

(1) *Rational competence* is an ability to make rational choices and judgments about oneself, which presupposes that the person has an adequately coherent set of beliefs that shapes his/her values, commitments and life plans in a consistent way. (This represents the "moderate" 50-80% range on the competency scale in Figure 2.1). Without consistency among an individual's beliefs, it is difficult for him/her to make rational decisions that reflect his/her innermost values and goals. If an individual's beliefs and values are inconsistent from situation to situation and decision to decision, his/her decisions will, in principle, be irrational (this reflects the "poor" 20-50% competency range in Figure 2.1). In short, to determine whether patient X will accept treatment Y, s(he) must have a moderately consistent set of values and beliefs in order to make an autonomous decision in favor of a medical treatment.

There are three dimensions of rational competence: (i) content; (ii) process; and (iii) outcome. Each of these dimensions are important for determining whether the decision was rationally made by the patient, and is therefore an important set of heuristics[3] that could be used by the physician to determine a patient's competence. A caveat is in order at this point. These three heuristics will not necessarily make it any easier for physicians to determine whether or not a patient is rationally competent. These dimensions take a substantial amount of time and patience to nurture and develop which requires open and honest communication between patient and physician.

(i) The *content* of rational competence is a reference to the beliefs that a person holds. If a patient is reasonable and rational, s(he) will act on the basis of the belief and value systems expressing decisions that are rational, and s(he) will reject all those beliefs and values that are irrational, inconsistent or incoherent. This is part of the revisionary process of the belief structures of every rational individual. The process requires reflection by the individuals and requires that s(he) assesses his/her inner self, so to speak, in order to determine whether his/her beliefs are consistent and rational, or inconsistent and irrational. (Such individuals usually fit between the 50%-80% range in Figure 2.1.) A reflective individual who has inconsistent beliefs may fit between the

Figure 2.1*

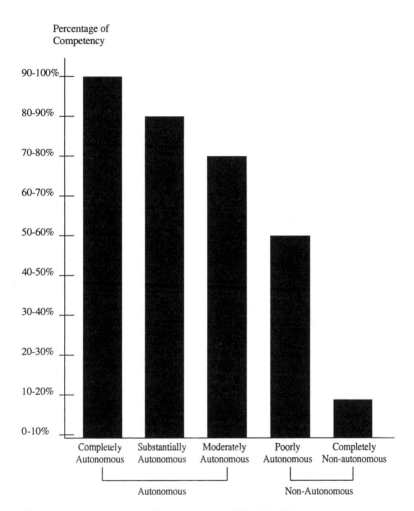

*The more autonomous a patient is, the more competent will be his/her decision. An autonomous individual has a consistent set of beliefs, values, and life goals. The more consistent their beliefs and life goals are, the more competent will a patient's decision be. There is a direct correlation between a patient's autonomy and his/her competency in making rational, consistent decisions.

50-80% range at say the 50-60% range of competency. The more capable a person is in replacing and/or modifying inconsistent beliefs with consistent ones, the more autonomous will his/her decisions be. This is achieved through an act of volition and self-reflexivity on the part of the patient. For instance, say a patient believes that one of his/her deeply held beliefs is to be honest, yet occasionally s(he) notices that s(he) lies. The rational person who becomes aware of this pattern of behavior would need to become more reflective and consciously try to stop lying until the habit ceases altogether.

(ii) The *process* of rational competence is closely related to the content. Through the process of rational competence, the individual forms judgments about his/her basic beliefs. When a patient is attempting to derive an informed consent, s(he) must "frame"[4] the information about a given medical treatment accurately. In short, in deciding about a medical treatment, the patient must decide in favor of the treatment by considering his/her life plans, goals and values and these must form a coherent unity. The choice of medical treatment must reflect the belief structures and values of the patient, and not be a hasty, unreflective choice. Such immediate reactions typically cannot count as rational judgments.

(iii) The *outcome* stage presupposes that the patient has not only rationally deliberated about the medical treatments, but is also ready to act on the basis of his/her choice. Many patients become intuitively aware which medical treatment would be the most rational to accept, yet make a decision in favor of a medical treatment in a way that is contrary to that initial intuition. A patient may rationally understand that s(he) should really undergo a particular medical treatment, say treatment A; yet, due to a weakness of the will or because of fear of the consequences of the treatment, s(he) will nevertheless opt for treatment B which is not in the patient's best interest. In this case, the outcome stage is less than competent, and is irrational. This type of case is all too common in medical practice, but the physician may sometimes have no immediate awareness that there is a difficulty.

It may be tempting to assume that if the content and process of rational competence is successful, then the outcome is not too important. In short, it might be tempting to assert the following formula:

Rational content + Rational process
= Rational competence

But this would be a misguided assertion. The most important aspect of rational competence focuses on a patient's ability to rationally act on the decision. Informed consent focuses primarily on the patient's ability to make rational decisions about the medical treatment that s(he) will undergo. This may take moral discipline for some patients to achieve due to the uncertainties that some diseases and medical treatments pose. However, a rational decision is still one that a patient acts on and not merely one s(he) simply decides to accept, but then fails to act on, which would be a kind of irrationality. To act in such a way would ultimately yield a non-autonomous consent.

(2) *Performance competence* is based on a person's capacity or capability to perform some task accurately and with minimal self-understanding. In the case of informed consent, this would translate into adequately consenting to a given medical treatment. By 'adequately consenting', is meant consenting on the basis of, or use of, some important principles of rationality and common sense and resulting from effective communication between patient and physician. Thus, the performance competence parameters of informed consent consists of at least:

(i) adequate understanding; and
(ii) adequate rational decision making.

Much more will be said about these two criteria for evaluating performance competence in the next two chapters. For the moment, a brief thumbnail sketch is in order to show how each is essential for performance competence.

(i) *Adequate understanding.* In order for a patient to understand a particular medical treatment(s), the physician must communicate all the medical treatments available and the risks and benefits involved in each treatment as well as the nature of each procedure. In the process, the physician must also communicate any possible complications with the medical procedures. This requires open discussion, so that the patient and physician could determine the side effects or complications of the treatments, how they will affect the patient, and which complications the patient can tolerate. Initially, the physician must communicate all the medical treatments to the patient which requires that the patient is capable of retaining them in memory to make an autonomous choice in favor of a medical treatment. The more capable a patient is of doing so, the more performance competent s(he) will be.

(ii) *Rational decision making.* Once a patient understands all the medical treatments available, s(he) must rationally assess them and decide in favor of a medical treatment, given the risks and benefits. Some treatments may be eliminated immediately, while others will be more difficult to eliminate. A patient might more readily agree to surgery than to mind-altering medications; thus, the option of surgery will be immediately rejected or vice versa. Whether the patient's decision is rationally competent is something that must be decided by the physician and patient. If the patient's decision is irrational, then it may have been 'framed' wrongly, influenced by biases such as fear of surgery, or fear and/or impatience with having one's mind affected by medication. When a patient biasely 'frames' the medical treatment, s(he) doesn't understand every aspect of the treatments, making the patient's decision irrational.[5]

The rational decision criterion of performance competence requires that the patient decide given the diagnostic treatment options that would be most reasonable for the patient to accept given the patient's particular medical situation. This is a minimal level where the patient's values, goals and life plans are not relevant although they will become progressively more important at a later stage of evaluation. Regrettably, many physicians never get beyond this minimal stage of patient performance evaluation. This is perhaps owing to several factors: (1) patient vulnerabilities (for example, the patient's lack of education, native intelligence, perspicuity, or a lack of rational decision making skills); (2) time constraints on the physician (and other health care professional(s); (3) lack of adequate communication between physician and patient due to personality clashes, or simply a physician's lack of interest in the patient; and (4) impatience on the part of the physician, who believes that such careful attention is beyond the call of duty as a physician.

Is the performance competence requirement as presented too demanding? The question must be answered negatively; what has been given so far is minimally necessary for achieving any properly informed consent. Some physicians may say that the understanding condition is much too demanding since while the physician must understand all of the medical treatments, the patient is not capable of comprehending them. This objection is more a criticism of the health profession than an assessment of the patient's capabilities for informed consent. Physicians must do whatever they can to assist the patients in understanding the medical procedures by using clear, unambiguous language that can be understood by most patients. If the patient fails to understand the treatments, s(he) will be unable to make a rational decision, and therefore his/her consent will be uninformed.

(3) *Reflective Competence* is perhaps the most important parameter of competence since it presupposes rational and performance competence. In evaluating a patient's reflective competence, the physician must determine whether the patient is capable of not merely retaining the information about the treatments, make a decision based on his/her beliefs, values, goals, and life plans, but the patient must also be able to determine whether the decision is consistent with his/her values, beliefs and goals. Reflective competence is a type of awareness that is essential to evaluate a patient's decision in favor of a medical treatment which requires stepping-back from the content of the decision. The process involved in stepping-back ensures that the patient makes a rational decision. Consider the following case.

A 37 year old woman goes in to see a physician for a medical exam complaining of heavy, long menstrual cycles that have been going on for six months. The patient is unsure of her exact diagnosis but knows that she is haemorrhaging during and between menstrual cycles which sometimes continues for weeks at a time. Initially, the physician believes that the problem will correct itself and prescribes minestrin, a birth control pill, to correct the situation. The problem does not however correct itself, and after a few months, the patient asks the general practitioner whether she can undergo an ultra sound of the uterus to detect if there are any growths such as fibroid tumours. The medical doctor reluctantly agrees saying that "it is normal for a woman her age to experience difficulties with her cycles".

The woman undergoes an ultra sound which shows that she has (in fact) several fibroid growths. Still the general practitioner insists that the problem could be treated through birth control pills, as long as the fibroids don't get larger. The condition doesn't correct itself, and the patient's condition seems to be getting worse. The general practitioner finally refers the patient to a gynaecologist who outlines several other medical treatments not yet mentioned by the general practitioner: (1) depo-provera; (2) a stronger birth control pill; (3) a medication to shrink the fibroids that may work, but has serious side effects, and a possible regrowth of fibroids a few months after taking the medication; and (4) a partial hysterectomy removing the uterus and cervix, but not the ovaries. The gynaecologist insists that the hysterectomy is the last resort after at least some, if not all, of the previous medical treatments have been tried.

The patient decides to forestall surgery and to try out the medications. First, she tries the depo-provera treatments; however, her condition worsens, and the woman now is severely anaemic and goes into the emergency department of the local hospital since she feels faint and weak. The general practitioner at the emergency department and the gynaecologist on call insist that surgery in now imminent. In order to stop the hemorrhaging, the woman is given a stronger birth control pill. The medication works as long s the woman is in bod, otherwise she still hemorrhages. The woman could still choose option (3) above. What should the woman do?

Obviously, the medically, rational treatment that the woman should choose is to undergo surgery as soon as possible. The medication only seems like a short-term cure, with a multitude of side effects that are debilitating to the woman's normal everyday functions. Let us postulate two possible solutions to the woman's dilemma by considering how two different women may have decided on a treatment in this situation.

Woman A: After reflection, she feels that she will undergo surgery and resolve her medical problem. The risks of the surgery are not as great as continuing to hemorrhage over a longer period of time. Thus, surgery is a short term hardship (the pain and suffering after surgery) for a long term gain (the resolution of the medical illness).

Woman B: After reflection, the woman feels that she should try option (3) to stop her hemorrhaging. She rationalizes her decision by saying that she will feel unfeminine when she has the surgery, and thus the hysterectomy should be the final option after she has tried everything else. It then turns out that the medication is a short term gain, for a long term hardship.

Which woman's decision is rational? It is quite obvious that given the woman's medical condition (her anaemia and hemorrhaging), it would be rational to have surgery sooner rather than later. Thus, Woman's B decision wasn't sufficiently reflective, since if she stepped back from her decision, it would become apparent to her that she shouldn't try having children at the age of 37 anyway, and she should improve her health situation as quickly as possible so that she doesn't risk getting even more ill.

During the process of reflective competence, the patient must determine whether his/her decision was free from biases or wishful thinking. A patient may have a bias against surgery because, for example, one of her parents died during surgery. If Woman B determines that her initial decision against surgery was biased in this way, and that surgery is the rational option given her medical situation, the patient must reconsider her initial decision and reassess her options. The patient may have high hopes that the medication will shrink her fibroids equally well, while in reality this may be wishful thinking and, surgery is the only certain way of permanently alleviating the medical condition. If the patient is competent and rationally reconsiders her decision and options, she would likely decide to undergo surgery despite her irrational fear that s(he) will die during surgery as one of her parents did a while ago. If the patient is rationally and reflectively less than rationally competent, however, the patient may not be able to go through an adequate process of critical self-assessment, and she will end up making a less than autonomous decision.

Sometimes, the reflectively incompetent patient might stubbornly stick to her initial decision and will be unable to reassess her decision since she will be caught within the "web of biases" that comprised her initial decision. This "web of biases" will blind the patient's reasoning capacity so that she will be convinced that her initial decision against surgery was the most rational decision. In the above case, the patient might opt for the drug treatment (Woman B) although it didn't have the same kind of promise of success as surgery. In addition, the patient would have to endure some debilitating side effects that may be detrimental to her quality of life in the future. However, Woman B still prefers to endure these hardships instead of opting for surgery due to her biases and fears of surgery. Thus, Woman B's decision is less than reflectively competent.

If a patient is less than reflectively competent, she will have a tendency towards making less than rational decisions. The biases leading to reflective incompetency and irrational decision making tend to complement and support one another. A reflectively incompetent patient simply considers the medical treatments disclosed in a hasty, unreflective way and is unable to step-back from the original decision to reassess the correctness of the initial judgment. Biased and irrational consent is the result and this is not informed consent. A rationally competent patient (on the other hand) would test, reassess and scrutinize her initial decision ensuring that no biases or false judgments were involved.

III. Competent, Incompetent and Wrong Decisions

There's a fine line between incompetent and competent decisions and mistaken or wrong decisions. Before proceeding to a definition of 'incompetent' and 'wrong' decisions, I will define the notion of 'competence'. Competency is a multi-layered and complex concept, one

that admits of degrees as well as grey areas, as is outlined in Figure 2.1.
A competent decision may be defined

> as a decision that is rational, reflective, and non-emotional that reflects a patient's own unique beliefs and values, goals and life plans.

The competent patient is capable of reflective deliberation, always critically assessing whether his/her original decision in favor of a medical treatment was rational, well-informed and not hasty. Thus, typically the competent patient has a mature, well-developed set of beliefs, values and goals, and a self-reflective attitude.

However. if a patient cannot make a properly rational decision about a medical treatment, her decision is less than competent or incompetent. An incompetent decision is defined as

> a decision that is inconsistent with the values, goals, beliefs, and life plans of the patient. (This is represented in the below 50% range in Figure 2.1.)

Such patients are often "borderline" cases who can make autonomous, competent decisions, given the help of the physicians or medical professionals who will guide the patient's thinking processes into making a competent decision. The initial discussions should provide an opportunity for physicians to determine the degree of a patient's competency, and also help the patient determine what his/her values and beliefs are. But even in this case, the physician should disclose all the medical treatments available to the patient, and reiterate them until they are adequately understood. If the patient can make a competent, autonomous decision, the patient will then be facilitated by the physician in a rational decision process.

In the case above, it is quite clear that Woman B's decision is incompetent since it was not based on her more deeply held beliefs and values, notwithstanding her fears and reservations about surgery (which all patients must endure). If a patient's decision does not adequately conform to the standard of reflection needed to critically assess his/her thinking processes, the patient's decision is less than competent and the physician must engage in further discussion with her to communicate as clearly as possible the consequences of his/her decision, and also to show that her thinking is less than rational. The discussion is not so much aimed at persuading him/her that s(he) decided wrongly, or on the basis of contra-indicated conditions, as to guide her to make the right decision by reviewing the medical treatments available yet a second (or even a third time if needed) until she understands how irrational her initial decision was. It may be fair to assume that after this second or third discussion, most patients (except the most vulnerable patients such as those who have no secondary or post-secondary education, or who are mentally challenged)[6] will make a rational and reflectively competent decision.

However, what if Woman B doesn't have any secondary or post-secondary schooling? What if on further examination, she lacks the self-knowledge and reflective skills to assess her initial decision? In this case, the onus would be on the medical professionals to help guide the woman's thinking processes step-by-step so that she could make a rational decision. More time and effort will be required for minimally competent patients to make rational decisions; however, the time must be expended otherwise the patient will not give an informed consent. Through the process of effective communication between patient and physician, the patient should be able to eventually make a rational and competent decision. On the autonomy-enhancing model, it is necessary that physicians make an effort to ensure competent decisions are made by patients since approximately thirty percent of patients are less than competent in one or all of the ways mentioned.

Roughly seventy percent of patients can be expected to give a competently informed consent according to the latest statistics. These figures are indeed startling. Any fully developed theory of informed consent must concern itself with the thirty percent that are less than competent or incompetent; these individuals must be guided in giving a rational and competent informed consent. Incompetent patients pose hardships and dilemmas for physicians since they usually have: (1) no coherent set of beliefs, values, commitments and life goals; (2) no coherent, rational thinking processes, in the sense of being consistent over time; (3) no well-developed sense of self, consistent character traits, and no sense of their likes and dislikes; (4) little ability to reflect on their values and goals; and (5) no retention skills needed to remember long lists of medical treatments. This makes the physician's responsibility for ensuring an informed consent much more difficult to achieve. However, despite these difficulties, the physician should still strive to ensure that such patients give an informed consent.

Lastly, let us consider wrong decisions. A wrong decision is defined as

a medically unacceptable decision based on past medical records and standard medical practice.

It makes little, if any, sense to categorize a wrong decision as non-autonomous, since wrong decisions can still be arrived at autonomously, albeit at a lower level of rationality. A wrong decision by the patient usually results when a patient "frames" the procedure irrationally. The decision is then typically an unreflective, emotional response to a medical treatment, one that is unreasoned and makes no coherent sense. It is also typically the case that no amount of reiteration and counseling of the procedures, and the risks and benefits of treatment will convince the patient to change his/her initial decision. An awareness of the consequences may hardly have any effect on the patient's decision, and s(he) will still blindly hold onto his/her wrong decision, and the physician will be unable to convince the patient to reassess his/her initial decision. Consider the following case.

Mr. Fontanez is an 82 year old who has been admitted to the medical service with a diagnosis of cancer of the pancreas which has metastasized (spread) to the liver, spleen, and bone. Upon admission, it is noted that Mr. Fontanez has gangrene of the foot and has already lost two toes. He is in considerable pain, with the daily cleaning and care of the foot causing more pain.

A surgeon is consulted and agrees with the attending physician that a partial amputation of the foot is the only hope for stopping the spread of the gangrene. Since the surgeon is the one who will do the procedure, he approaches Mr. Fontanez for consent. He explains the procedure, tells Mr. Fontanez why it is necessary, and then asks him to sign the form consenting to the operation. Mr. Fontanez refuses to sign. The surgeon carefully explains the consequences of not having the operation (continued pain and spread of the disease). However, Mr. Fontanez still refuses, saying, "No, leave me alone and let me die in peace."[7]

Mr. Fontanez's decision is wrong because it is medically contra-indicated for the patient to give up hope of having his gangrene treated even though the chances of curing pancreatic cancer are slim. The physician cannot change the patient's irrational decision, which seems suicidal since he prefers to die rather than have his leg amputated. No rational patient would make such a hasty, less than rational choice. The patient is in denial about the facts of his disease, and the consequences of his decision.

IV. Tests for Competency

There are three well known tests[8] available for determining whether a patient is competent. It should be pointed out, however, that these tests presuppose that the patients were usually competent to make rational decisions, and that illness, medication, age and so on only circumstantially or incidentally affected their rational capabilities and competence level. If this is not the case, such as with the severely psychologically incompetent patients, these tests do not apply. The three tests of competency are: (1) the outcome competency test; (2) the status competency test; and (3) the function competency test. All three tests are conducted on patients presumed to be partially incompetent after some initial observations of their rational decision making skills.[9]

(1) *The outcome competency test* determines whether a patient's decision for treatment is in synchrony with other medical decisions in similar circumstances. If a patient's decision seems irrational in comparison to other patient's decisions of the same or similar medical situation, his/her decision can be deemed incompetent. This test is, by itself, insufficient since it fails to seriously take the uniqueness of an

individual patient into consideration; the test presupposes that the patient is not fully competent to make his/her own decisions and thus his/her autonomy could be questioned. The number of successful times a particular treatment has been used for an illness does not make it right for every patient to accept.

(2) *The Status competency test* determines whether a patient's mental and/or physical status may affect his/her capability for rational and competent decisions. Some of the features of status are health related factors such as the patient's medical situation (i.e., whether a patient has been in long-term care such as an institution or hospital setting), the age of the patient (i.e., old age or immaturity may affect a patient's decisions), the prolonged use of certain medications that may affect a patient's ability to think clearly, and a patient's education level. Health professionals may sometimes find it especially difficult to convince older patients that they should not give up on life and accept treatment, even if it only seems to prolong their life by just a few years. If, in addition, the older patient's illness causes constant pain, s(he) will most likely not want to prolong life by undergoing further treatment. The decision against treatment is, in principle, irrational. The test is devised to categorized such decisions as incompetent. In this case, proxy consent may become necessary.

(3) *The function competency test* is concerned with the rationality of the patient's decision making skills about a particular medical treatment. It cannot be assumed that all patients are either rational or irrational, or competent or incompetent, decision makers. There are many grey areas in a patient's decision making; some individuals may fail to make decisions uniformly. Instead, competence in decision making is a matter of degree. Most patients make at least some rational decisions which are competent, while the rationality of other decisions may be questioned. It is also a well known psychological fact that most irrational decisions are made when people feel especially vulnerable and insecure which is common when a patient enters a hospital with an unknown diagnosis, feeling pain, weak and distressed. Most patients would find it difficult to make competent decisions on the spur of the moment since they feel alienated, so to speak, from their values, beliefs, and life plans due to illness. If the patient has ample

time to reflect, s(he) will usually make a competent decision in favor of a medical treatment.

If a patient fails one of the three competency tests, the patient will be deemed incompetent, and diminished competency results in restricted autonomy. Therefore, the patient will be unable to make a rational decision about treatment, and as a result, s(he) will not achieve an informed consent. It may be possible for a physician to repeat the medical treatments and guide the patient's reasoning so that a competent decision will result. This method of reiteration is sometimes successful since many patients find it difficult to initially understand and retain medical information they have never encountered prior to becoming ill.

If a patient is still deemed incompetent, proxy consent becomes necessary. Proxy consent "is consent given by a secondary consenter on behalf of the primary consenter."[10] The primary consenter (the patient) is placed in the care of a secondary consenter (surrogate) to make decisions on the patient's behalf, and to give consent to treatment. There are several obvious difficulties with proxy consent: (1) How could another person's judgment be substituted for the patient's? No other person (no matter how closely connected to the patient) can ever know with complete certainty how the patient would decide if s(he) was competent. The patient's values, beliefs, and goals could only be experienced and understood coherently by the patient himself/herself. No outside source (surrogate) can be well enough informed to make such decisions on behalf of the patient, since autonomy is not transferable from person to person. The result is that the surrogate can only give mere consent, and not informed consent for a medical treatment. In short, proxy consent cannot be informed consent because we can never have a complete grasp of another person's beliefs, values, and goals. The second or third party consenter must inevitably project his/her values onto the values of the primary consenter, which usually results in further difficulties, and may lead to non-informed consent. What is essential on the autonomy-enhancing model is that a patient's decision for treatment be based on his/her own individual and unique values, goals, beliefs and life plans. Thus, it is imperative that if at all possible (with the exception of patients in a coma and the severely mentally incompetent), patients must make their own decision in favor of a medical treatment.

Notes

1. Morreim, Haavi. "Three Concepts of Patient Competence". *Theoretical Medicine*, 4 (1983), 232.
2. This threefold distinction of competence originated in Haavi Moreim's article as referenced in footnote 1.
3. Heuristics are rules of thumb or guidelines for a decision that can be used by patients and physicians.
4. The "framing" effect will be defined and discussed below under the heading of "rational decision making".
5. More will be said about rational decision making in chapter 5.
6. Such individuals are excluded from consideration here since they fall below the 50 percent level of competency outlined in Figure 2.1 above. As the figure shows, such patients cannot give a properly informed consent.
7. This case was taken from Richard Wright's *Human Values in Health Care: The Practice of Ethics.* New York: McGraw Hill Book Company, 1987), p. 106.
8. The impetus for this discussion is taken from Richard Wright's *Human Values in Health Care*, p. 110ff.
9. Richard Wright argues (p. 107) in *Human Values in Health Care: The Practice of Ethics,* that only the outcome test and status test presumes that the patient is incompetent. I would argue that all three tests presume patient incompetence; however, a defence of this is beyond the scope of this chapter, as it would lengthen an already long chapter.
10. Richard Wright, *Human Values in Health Care: The Practice of Ethics,* p. 108.

Chapter 3

Physician Disclosure of Medical Treatments

Physician-disclosure is an important first condition for achieving an informed consent and for the nurturing of an effective physician-patient relationship.[1] The notion of disclosure has, however, gone through a multitude of structural changes over the past three decades or so. Up to the 1960's, physicians were reluctant to disclose any detailed information about the patient's diagnosis since they assumed that:[2] (1) the patient did not want to know; (2) the patient wouldn't understand the information anyway, so why spend time and effort disclosing it; (3) the physician always knows what is in the best interest of the patient making it unnecessary to get the patient involved and further complicate matters; (4) the physician has both the authority and medical knowledge to prescribe certain treatments to the patient, who has an obligation to accept treatment; and (5) patients were previously uninformed about their health, making it rather tedious, costly, and time-consuming for physicians to discuss the medical treatments in detail. At present, this knowledge gap between patient and physician has been greatly reduced since medical knowledge is much more available to lay persons through television learning channels, medical self-help books and the internet. The 1960's idea of informed consent (as outlined above) relies heavily on the traditional harm-avoidance model that focuses on the physician as a medical authority who makes decisions in favor of a patient's medical treatment. This chapter focuses on the kind of disclosure that is necessary for a patient to achieve an informed consent on the autonomy-enhancing model.

38   *A New Paradigm For Informed Consent*

I. Two Standards of Physician-disclosure

There are two common standards of disclosure[3] that physicians have used over the decades:

(1) The 'professional practice' standard; and
(2) The 'reasonable person' standard.

Both of these standards have had an impact on physicians' views about disclosure, especially about how much, or how little information is to be disclosed to the patient about his/her diagnosis and prognosis. Physicians are still in fundamental disagreement about which standard of disclosure should be adopted to ensure an informed consent, and there has been no universal adoption of one standard over another. Regardless of which standard a particular physician uses, it is generally conceded that it is a physician's professional duty (since the 1980's at any rate) to give patients adequate information about their treatments (and the risks and benefits) to ensure that the patient is substantially informed about his/her medical options.

(1) *The 'Professional Practice' standard* is the traditional, paternalistic model of disclosure which focuses on the physician as the final decision maker with respect to which treatment is in the patient's best interest. This standard relies heavily on the Hippocratic tradition in which the physician is viewed as the person who authoritatively and paternalistically makes a decision about a particular treatment, while the patient passively and non-reflectively accepts the physician's decision. This standard stresses the principle of beneficence while at the same time undermining the principle of autonomy.

Disclosure under this standard is minimal since the communication between the physician and patient takes the form of a prescription: "In order to cure your illness/disease, I suggest you undergo treatment X or medication Y". The patient then accepts the treatment suggested by the physician since it is assumed that the physician has evaluated and assessed all the treatments available to the patient. But how can a physician who communicates so little to the patient know what is in the patient's best interest? The medical knowledge that a physician has cannot possibly be equated with the personal knowledge that is required for information about a patient's beliefs and values that are necessary for assessing the treatments and for determining what is in the patient's best interest. A physician needs both medical knowledge and the personal knowledge of the patient in order to accurately determine which treatment is suitable for a particular patient.

On the autonomy-enhancing model, this kind of paternalism is unacceptable since it undermines a patient's autonomy and self-determination. Since disclosure is not required on this standard, informed consent cannot be achieved. In order for an informed consent to be achieved, physicians must disclose information about all the risks and benefits of treatments, and patients must make an autonomous decision on the basis of the medical information which is consistent with their beliefs and values. No physician can ever have such knowledge about his/her patient without extended communication with the patient, suggesting a kind of partnership that allows both parties to fill in gaps in their knowledge. The patient lacks medical knowledge while the physician lacks the patient's personal knowledge. On the traditional view, such gaps are not relevant to giving an informed consent, while on the autonomy-enhancing model, such gaps are not only relevant, but must be transcended.

(2) *The 'reasonable person' standard* of disclosure focuses on the information about the medical treatments that are necessary for a patient to understand the risks, benefits, and harms of the treatment. On this view, a physician has a duty to disclose any information about the treatments that a "reasonable person" would require to make a substantially understood, rational decision. The physician and patient must enter into a relationship of open, honest communication so that they can both form an hypothesis about the best medical treatment. The patient, however, must ultimately decide which medical treatment is in his/her best interest. The physician must respect the patient's autonomy by encouraging the patient to participate in his/her own decision making in favor of a particular medical procedure.

The "reasonable person" standard is a considerable improvement over the "professional practice" standard since an *informed* consent is achievable. The protection of the patient's autonomy is the primary purpose of informed consent. Complete disclosure of information about the medical treatments is absolutely necessary if the physician is to respect the patient's autonomy and ensure that s(he) will give an informed consent. Otherwise, the patient's autonomy will be undermined and an informed consent will not be achieved. It is morally wrong to perform any medical treatment without a patient's expressed, autonomous permission. The passive, non-autonomous acceptance of treatment by the patient that is based solely on the physician's decision, as is the case on the "professional practice" standard, is unacceptable.

An important aspect of the "reasonable person" standard is not only the disclosure of the treatments but a disclosure of *all* the known risks of treatment, even if they are remote and may only happen infrequently. The following case makes this point clearer (Gillon 1994, 437):

> In 1954 a young freelance broadcaster developed a toxic goitre. A general practitioner asked a consultant physician at a London teaching hospital to see her, and he advised that a partial thyroidectomy as an alternative to medical treatment was the better course. The operation was performed by a surgeon who was asked by the patient whether there was any risk to her voice. He told her that there was none. Unfortunately, after the operation her voice was weak. There was paralysis of the left vocal chord from damage to the laryngeal nerve which passes behind the thyroid gland. Her complaint against the consultant physician was that he had, according to her, negligently advised that the operation involved no risk to her voice, and that had she known there was any risk she would have chosen treatment rather than the operation."4

In the above case, the physician is morally and legally culpable since he told the patient that there was no risk to her voice with the particular treatment when in fact there was a risk. On the autonomy-enhancing model developed in the book, all the known, relevant risks should have been disclosed and not only the most probable risks. From the fact that the patient had a career as a freelance broadcaster, the information about the risk to her voice was clearly relevant and should have been disclosed by the surgeon. Thus, the surgeon violated the patient's right to self-determination and autonomy by not disclosing this information, and her consent for the procedure was not informed.

II. Paradigm Shift in the Notion of Disclosure

In the early 1970's, there was a fundamental shift in physician's attitudes towards disclosure and this marks a paradigm shift in patient consent. This paradigm shift is still presently molding itself into a unified standard. It is difficult to understand what the ultimate purpose of patient consent to treatment could have been before the early 1960's when medical decisions were made paternalistically and prescriptively. The procedure for patient consent during the 1960's was relatively simple, but it was not informed nor autonomous according to the autonomy-enhancing model, since it consisted of: (1) a patient consulting a physician about a medical problem; (2) the physician prescribing a treatment that s(he) has chosen without consulting the patient; and (3) the patient either accepting or refusing the treatment prescribed. No alternative treatments were communicated to the patient; as far as the patient was aware, there was only one possible treatment – i.e., the one the physician was prescribing. The obvious conclusion is that consent in the 1960's was not informed consent, since the treatment was not autonomously chosen by the patient. In terms of the new human rights movement, physicians before the 1960's were violating the patient's human rights.

Thus, consent for a medical treatment had to evolve into an informed consent for the patient's right to self-determination and for autonomy to be respected. Physicians were initially[5] strongly reluctant to invite their patients into the decision-making process of considering the various treatments had available to the patient. It took a decade for physicians to begin to accept this ideal of informed consent.[6] The reluctance was mainly due to the physicians insisting that there be no intrusiveness of their medical practice by those who lack medical expertise. Specifically, physicians believed that the medical practice was autonomous and not to be intruded upon by patients. This attitude on the part of physicians began to change when they realized that a patient's illness affects the whole person, and not just the body. Thus, the patient must be involved in the decision process to choose the best medical treatment available.

Nine percent of physicians in a survey in the early 1970's, reported that they did not disclose the details of the patient's diagnosis (see Table 3.1). In 1978, only two percent of the physicians still failed to disclose information about treatment, while 98% did in fact disclose the medical treatments available to the patient. The reasons for this sudden change in a physician's attitude towards disclosure are difficult to precisely pin down. It is quite possible that the focus on human rights at the time created more concern for individuality and moral autonomy. The authority-based structure of medicine in the 1960's had to change in order to accommodate the concerns of the human rights movement. It became quite clear that it was morally inappropriate for physicians to treat patients non-autonomously, i.e., by simply prescribing treatments that the patients must accept without any further consultation on the part of the physician.

III. Difficulties With Disclosure

Once disclosure became a fairly acceptable practice for physicians by the late 1970's, certain difficulties came to the surface. Some of the problems of disclosure[7] discovered were as follows:

1. Should physicians *disclose the details of diseases*, such as cancer, that may ultimately terminate a patient's life, in spite of the painful treatments and discomfort that the patient must endure which may only prolong life by a few years.
2. *How much information should the physician disclose to* patient before an informed consent can be given?
3. How much *technical/medical jargon* must be explained by the physician in order that patients fully understand the physician's descriptions of the treatments?
4. Should the *intentional use of manipulators* be used to persuade patients to accept a particular treatment?

1. *Disclosure of details of the disease.* Some physicians argue against disclosure since they have observed that a negative prognosis about a disease may cause adverse health consequences such as depression, anxiety, or irrational fears, making the patient feel hopeless.

Table 3.1*

Year	Percentage	Description
1953	69%	– Physicians never told patients the details of diagnosis
	31%	– Disclosed information of the diagnosis
1960	22%	– Physicians *never* told patients the details of diagnosis
	16%	– Physicians *always* informed the patient
1961	90%	– Physicians generally failed to inform patients of diagnosis
	10%	– Physicians informed patients
1970	9%	– Physicians said they never told patients of their diagnosis
	25%	– Physicians always told the patient
1975	98%	– Physicians reported that it was general policy to tell the patients of diagnosis
	2%	– Physicians failed to report the diagnosis to patients

*The statistics for this table were taken from Richard Goldenberg's essay "Disclosure of Information to Adult Cancer Patients" in Richard Wright *Human Value in Health Care: The Practice of Ethics* (New York: McGraw Hill Book Company, 1987).

The result is that the patient tends to make irrational decisions about the treatments available. It is for this reason that some physicians still refrain from disclosing all the details about medical diagnoses to their patients. Is it morally obligatory for physicians to disclose a negative prognosis, despite the possible psychological difficulties that a negative prognosis may cause for some patients?

On the autonomy-enhancing model, it is *never* morally permissible for physicians to not disclose information about the diagnosis, prognosis or the medical treatments, along with the risks and benefits of each treatment. Failure to do so undermines a patient's right to self-determination as well as the patient's autonomy, thereby making it impossible for a patient to give a properly informed consent. For properly informed consent, the physician must disclose all the relevant information of the diagnosis to the patient, regardless of whether the information is positive or negative, and the patient must decide for him/herself whether or not to endure a particular treatment. In the case of cancer patients, for instance, physicians have a duty to disclose all the known alternatives as well as the possibility that after the treatment the symptoms of the disease may return. If the patient, for instance, refuses chemotherapy because of its negative side effects and the likelihood that his/her quality of life will be greatly diminished, the physician (given the circumstances) may have to allow the patient to die without treatment, assuming that the patient's decision was reflective and autonomous. Many patients that are diagnosed with certain cancers, such as lymph cancer, understand that they may not only live for more than three or four years after treatment. Most physicians prescribe chemotherapy to patients with lymph cancer, but some patients refuse treatment owing to the inevitability of death, and the pain and discomfort that is involved. Patients that refuse chemotherapy typically are concerned for the quality of life, and may believe in living with dignity. If such conditions do not prevail, they prefer to not endure chemotherapy and be left to die.

Whether it is rational for a cancer patient to refuse chemotherapy in this situation is a question that is best left until the discussion on rational decision making in Chapter 5. For the present, it is important to emphasize that despite the possible drawbacks of complete disclosure of treatment(s) for certain cancer and chronic disease patients, the physician still has a moral duty to disclose all the information about a patient's disease despite its negative effects, and thereby treat the patient as an autonomous agent. A patient's illness may make him/her feel helpless and vulnerable; however, the patient must make his/her own decisions, and thus physicians must communicate all the medical treatments available so that the patient will be able to give an autonomous consent for a medical treatment. Consider the following case:

> Barbara Wainwright, a 57-year old mother of two, was admitted to the hospital to rule out obstructive cancer of the colon. While the tests are being processed, Barbara's husband and children meet the doctor and ask her not to tell Barbara if the results are positive. They tell the doctor that Barbara fears cancer very much, and they believe she would become extremely upset and depressed, and give up all desire to live. "Don't tell her", they say. "It will be too hard on her". The physician is unhappy with this request because she believes in giving patients information about their diagnosis. The family insists, however, that Barbara not be told, so the physician reluctantly agrees. The tests come back positive; but when Barbara asks about them, the physician says: "The tests are inconclusive, but don't worry, you'll do just fine."[8]

This example is an instance of how physicians may sometimes be distracted by manipulative relatives to undermine a patient's right to autonomous decision making. The physician may have been operating on the harm-avoidance model of informed consent, and believed that if she told Barbara about her cancer, she would lose hope and her medical condition would become even worse. Even if the physician knows first hand through extensive conversation with the patient that she would react negatively to a positive result on the test, the physician still has a moral duty to disclose this information on the autonomy-enhancing model. If anything, the physician should try to prepare the patient psychologically for the honest disclosure. The physician's priority must be to his/her patient and not to her relatives unless there is a strong reason to suppose that she is incompetent to face the facts about her prognosis; but this is unlikely from the details of the case.

2. *How much information should the physician disclose to the patient?* Physicians are sometimes anxious about what kinds of information and how much information should be disclosed to the patient. At the very minimum, the physician must disclose the following:

(1) an explanation of all the known and relevant medical procedures that can be performed to alleviate the illness and pain;
(2) the purpose(s) of the various treatments;
(3) a description of the risks that may be involved in each of the treatments;
(4) an assessment of the pain and risks and how they may affect a particular patient given his/her age, tolerance of pain and endurance level;
(5) a description of the benefits of each treatment;
(6) an assessment of which benefits are most relevant to the patient given his/her beliefs, values, goals and life plans;
(7) a specified time when a patient's questions will be answered by the physician; and
(8) a statement by the physician that the patient can withdraw consent for any or all of the procedures.

Most of these aspects of disclosure are fairly straightforward to achieve except for the first one. How many different procedures is it necessary for a physician to disclose to the patient? Clearly, it depends on the patient: some patients will want to know all the risks and benefits involved, including the possible negative risks, even if they may be remote. Other patients may prefer to know only some of the more relevant details of treatment. Ideally, the patient should specify his/her personal preferences of disclosure since without precise instructions, the physician has a moral responsibility to disclose all the information about the alternative procedures and this may be time consuming. In any case, physicians should not try to determine what is in the patient's best interest without first consulting the patient.

The amount of information the physician discloses about alternative treatments may overreach a patient's retention capacity, and thus adversely influence his/her decision-making capabilities in favor of a medical treatment. Psychological research emphasizes the limitation of a normal person's retention ability to be 7 ± 2 bits of information at any one time in normal circumstances.[9] Given medical hardships, pain and the influence of medications on the patient's memory capacity, the above standard may be further diminished. The amount by which memory may be diminished obviously varies from patient to patient, and physicians should have an intuition into their patient's memory capacity. There are at least two ways that the physician may circumvent such retention difficulties:

(i) *A multi-staged process of disclosure.* In order to ensure that the patient doesn't reach cognitive saturation, the physician may opt to discuss the patient's treatments and their risks and benefits over several scheduled sessions, rather than one long, two or three hour, session. A single session may not be sufficient for adequate understanding of the information disclosed; disclosure is a *process* which takes time and effort. For instance, each of the sessions should be no longer than twenty minutes in duration since patients cannot retain information for any longer. The physician should schedule four or more sessions (depending on the disease or illness) with a patient to disclose all the medical treatments and to ensure that the patient makes an autonomous decision on the bases of such disclosure. This process helps patients digest all the treatments available and reflect on each of them carefully in order to make a rational, well-balanced decision in favor of a treatment. The more complicated the details of the treatment, the more time should be devoted by the physician to discuss the treatment alternatives, and the more time may be necessary for a patient to reflect adequately about the treatments' risks and benefits. Also, the more mentally and physically incapacitated a patient is due to illness or medication, the more time is required for the patient to make an autonomous decision.

(ii) *Reiteration.* Another way of circumventing the patient's possible retention difficulties is for the physician to reiterate all the available medical treatments and the risks and benefits. For some patients, all the unfamiliar medical jargon may further confuse them and make them unable to make a substantially informed consent. The process of reiteration need not take a substantial amount of additional time; the physician could at least expect that some of the information initially relayed to the patient will be recalled, making it easier for the patient to understand the information. However, it may still be desirable to have several reiteration sessions, depending on the patient. The level of a patient's understanding usually has an impact on whether s(he) retains all the details of the treatments the first time they are presented. If time constraints are an issue, physicians could have nurses or other medical professionals reiterate the details of the treatments, and give the patient a sufficient amount of time to absorb the information.

(3) *Technical/Medical Jargon.* Physicians should disclose the medical treatments in a non-technical way so that patients can adequately understand the information disclosed. This is possible despite protestations by some physicians that this is difficult to achieve. Physicians seem to communicate quite clearly with one another about new and common medical treatments since they are familiar with the medical jargon. It is unrealistic for physicians to expect their patients to understand such terminology. If some medical jargon is unavoidable in the explanation of certain medical procedures, these terms should be explained to patients using non-medical terminology to ensure that the information will be understood. If a physician fails to take these steps, the patient will not be able to give an informed consent since s(he) will not substantially understand the treatment(s) and their risks and benefits.

Having said all of this about disclosure, a caveat is in order. Although on the autonomy-enhancing model developed in the book, the physician has a duty to disclose all of the relevant details of the treatment alternatives to his/her patient, full and total disclosure is impossible due to the psychological limitations of patients, and the physicians lack of complete knowledge of the patient's personal values, beliefs, goals and life plans. Physicians may not even know all of the treatments that are available to the patient. However, it is fair, I think, to insist that physicians have a duty to disclose as much of the relevant information that they are aware of about the treatments available. There are, of course, gray areas in characterizing precisely what constitutes the relevant aspects of a treatment. The 'relevant information' criterion may vary from patient to patient and from physician to physician, making it difficult for the physician to determine, without detailed investigations and discussions, what information must be disclosed to a particular patient.

4. *Intentional use of Manipulators.* Another difficulty with disclosure is the intentional use of manipulators to persuade patients to accept a particular treatment in lieu of another one that the patient may have chosen. If a physician deliberately attempts to influence a patient's decision in favor of a treatment based on the physician's preferences, this stifles the process of understanding the medical treatments, and is a way of coercing the patient into agreeing with the physician. Such deliberate influences by the physician are common but they undermine a patient's ability to make an autonomous decision; thus, an informed consent cannot be achieved by the patient.

On the autonomy-enhancing model, any such deliberate influences are to be avoided. Physicians are under an obligation to disclose the medical treatments as unbiasedly as possible, and then assess and evaluate the treatments in consultation with the patient. Difficulties arise when physicians try to simultaneously disclose and evaluate the medical procedures. An assessment of the medical procedures is complex to achieve and should follow the disclosure of the medical treatments. In order to adequately assess the treatments according to the patient's personal preferences, the patient must:

(1) *Understand* the information disclosed;
(2) Make a *rational decision* that is unbiased and framed properly and adequately;)
(3) Be *reflective* about whether the patient's choice is genuinely what s(he) deeply thinks is appropriate -- in a sense this stage is the patient's testing of his/her original hypothesis. Is this really what the patient believes is genuinely coherent with his/her life plans, goals and values? and
(4) Engage in *effective communication* with the physician.[10]

Many physicians believe that 'adequate disclosure' is sufficient for a patient to achieve an informed consent. I argue that adequate disclosure is incomplete to achieve an informed consent, since it reinforces the traditional, paternalistic professional practice standard of informed consent. Thus, much more than adequate disclosure is necessary for achieving an informed consent.

IV. Substantial, Adequate and Incomplete Disclosure

There are three distinct kinds of disclosure:[11] (1) substantial; (2) adequate; and (3) incomplete.[12] Of the three kinds of disclosure, 'adequate disclosure' is the most problematic since there are gray areas which make it highly unlikely that an autonomous, informed decision can be made by any patient. This is especially the case to the right of the center mark of 'adequate disclosure' in Figure 3.2. To the left of center, it is highly probable that the decision a patient has made may be autonomous and informed. To the right of center, it is highly probable that the decision made is less than autonomous, and non-informed. However, the distinction between the "left" and "right" of center is sometimes difficult to fully determine with a high degree of certainty. To eliminate such uncertainty, I opt for 'substantial disclosure" in which the parameters of autonomous, informed consent can be predicted with much more certainty by physicians.

Thus, on the basis of the autonomy-enhancing model developed here, it is argued that "substantial disclosure" is a necessary and sufficient condition for ensuring with certainty that an informed consent is achieved. "Substantial disclosure" will be defined for the present purposes as:

> a communication by the physician, taking into account the patient's unique personal beliefs, values and life plans, of all the known and relevant alternatives of treatment and their possible risks and benefits in a non-technical manner such that the patient can understand the alternatives and is enabled to give an informed consent, based on a reflection of his/her deeply held values, goals, beliefs, and life plans.

In this way, the physician respects his/her patient's autonomy by ensuring that an autonomous decision is made in favor of a medical treatment. The physician has a duty to provide a *substantial* disclosure of the treatments available to ensure that the patient will make an autonomous decision. 'Adequate disclosure' and 'incomplete disclosure' can be distinguished as follows.

Figure 3.2

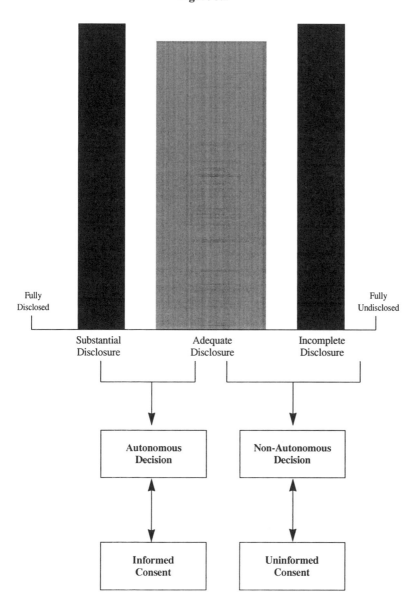

'Adequate disclosure' may still result in an autonomous decision about a medical treatment, although what counts as 'autonomous' is minimal. Autonomous decisions are made when one can choose from a list of medical treatments. The patient, however, has no knowledge of all the relevant treatment options available to him/her.

'Incomplete disclosure' is characterized as an ineffective disclosure of the medical treatments to the patient that conceals some or most of the important and relevant details of treatment from the patient, and makes it impossible for the patient to give an autonomous consent. This minimalist disclosure is advocated by traditional, paternalistic physicians who chose the treatment options for the patient. The one or two medical treatments are chosen by the physician without the patient's knowledge. This minimal disclosure relies on the paternalistic professional standard of disclosure. I argue that only 'substantial disclosure' can yield autonomous decisions.

It is quite obvious why 'adequate' and 'incomplete' disclosure is insufficient for achieving an informed consent. In order for a patient to give an informed consent, the physician must disclose all the treatment alternatives, and all the risks and benefits in order for the patient to give a reflective and autonomously informed consent. 'Adequate disclosure' is insufficient since the physician is still operating on the harm-avoidance model of informed consent by choosing the alternatives on behalf of the patient without consulting him/her. This is inappropriate for achieving an informed consent. 'Inadequate disclosure' is completely insufficient for achieving an informed consent since it solely relies on the authority and expertise of the physician in deciding which medical treatment the patient should undergo. It then follows that the patient simply agrees to the treatment but does not consent to it much less give an informed consent. Thus, 'substantial disclosure' by the physician is one of the preconditions for a patient to achieve an informed consent.

Notes

1. There are two kinds of disclosure recognized in medical contexts: (1) a disclosure of all the alternatives and their risks and benefits; and (2) a disclosure of medical diagnoses. Although these two kinds of disclosure may structurally vary, I will refer to both of them as general disclosure since the key issues of both kinds of disclosure seem to collapse into each other.
2. These statistics are formulated in Table 1 below.
3. These two standards of disclosure are mentioned by Michael Henderson in his essay "Risk and Doctor-Patient Relationship" in *Principles of Health Care Ethics* by Raanan Gillon, p. 435-444.
4. This case is presented in Michael Henderson's essay "Risk and Doctor-Patient Relationship" in *Principles of Health Care Ethics* by Raanan Gillon, p. 437.
5. Some physicians are still reluctant to treat their patients as partners in deciding in favor of a medical treatment alternative.
6. See Table 3.1. The statistics for this table were taken from Richard Goldenberg's essay "Disclosure of Information to Adult Cancer Patients" in Richard Wright *Human Values in Health Care: The Practice of Ethics* (New York: McGraw Hill Book Company, 1987).
7. The problems with disclosure is discussed by Richard Goldenberg "Disclosure of information to Adult Cancer Patients" in Richard Wright's *Human Values in Health Care: The Practice of Ethics* (New York: McGraw Hill Book Company, 1987), p. 114.
8. Richard Wright, *Human Values in Health Care: The Practice of Ethics* (New York: McGraw Hill Book Company, 1987), p. 114.
9. This psychological research is presented by G.A. Miller, "The Magical Number Seven, Plus or Minus Two: Some Limits on our Capacity for Processing Information". *Psychological Review*, (1956) (63), 81-87.
10. Each of these featues of assessment will be examined in subsequent chapters.
11. See Figure 3.2 below for an illustration of these three distinctions.
12. I will not deal with either 'full disclosure' or 'full concealment' since informed consent isn't an issue at either extreme At the level of 'full disclosure', the patient presumably has a complete knowledge of his/her values, beliefs, life goals and so on and can make a rational and autonomous decision that is completely reflective of his personal attributes. There are very few, if any, patients that are capable of such coherence among their beliefs. However, if such individuals were conceivable, an informed

consent would be achieved effortlessly each and every time; there would be no gray areas whatsoever. A similar case can be made out for 'full concealment' in that there is no uncertainty as to the status of psychologically incompetent patients making decisions. In this case, the patient has no coherent set of beliefs, values, or life plans to rely on to make an autonomous decision about a medical intervention that is reflective of his/her person. Thus, the consent given in such circumstances will always be non-autonomous and non-informed, and an informed consent cannot be achieved under any circumstances.

Chapter 4

Understanding Between Patient and Physician

A second important subjective condition for achieving informed consent is the degree and accuracy of the patient's understanding of the medical treatments and risks disclosed by the physician about the available treatments. Understanding may be characterized as the patient's assimilation of the information about the medical treatments. The criteria of understanding is complex since it involves the psychological and intellectual idiosyncrasies unique to each individual patient. Each patient's degree and level of understanding must be assessed by the physician in order to determine how much medical information a particular patient can absorb about the treatments and whether the patient will require extra attention such as reiteration or other kinds of memory aids in order to substantially understand the treatments. There are four conditions for ensuring that a patient substantially understands the treatments disclosed by the physician: (1) open communication; (2) shared understanding; (3) relevancy of information disclosed; and (4) sparing use of medical jargon by physician. Before discussing these four conditions, I will distinguish three kinds of understanding, one of which is essential to informed consent.

I. "Substantial Understanding", "Adequate Understanding" and "Inadequate Understanding"

It will be my contention in this chapter that a patient must achieve a "substantial understanding" of the treatments available in order to achieve an informed consent. This doesn't mean that the patient must *completely understand* all the details about the treatments available in order to achieve an informed consent. This would be too unrealistic to demand and impossible to achieve since physicians can never disclose all the information about a medical procedure and its options, and neither can patients fully understand all the medical intricacies of the treatments. Neither is a patient who is fully ignorant or even minimally ignorant of the treatments capable of achieving an informed consent. Such minimal ignorance may be referred to as "inadequate understanding" meaning that the patient understands very few of the medical treatments that are disclosed by the physician. Further, a patient who only adequately understands the medical treatments disclosed is also lacking the necessary comprehension of detail that is necessary to achieve an informed consent.[1] "Adequate understanding" consists of substantially understanding the medical treatments disclosed by the physician. The patient is not part of the process of choosing the relevant medical treatments; the physician simply chooses the treatments on the patient's behalf. Since both "adequate" and "inadequate" understanding result in non-autonomous consent, physicians must aim at achieving a "substantial" understanding, the detailed process of which will be explicated below.

II. The Four Conditions for "Substantial Understanding"

On the autonomy-enhancing model, a patient must "substantially" understand the treatments in order to give an informed consent. A substantial amount of detailed information must be disclosed by the physician in order for the patient to substantially understand the treatments. Some of the medical information that must be disclosed is as follows:

Figure 4.1

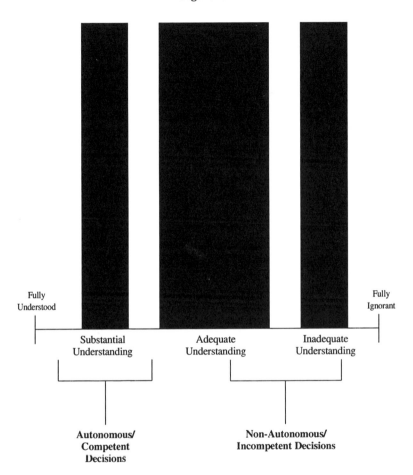

(1)   all the risks and benefits involved in each treatment;
(2)   the statistics about the success rate of each procedure based on past records;
(3)   the pain and hardship that is involved for each treatment;
(4)   the amount of time that will be necessary for the patient to convalesce after each treatment;
(5)   a detailed description of the procedure that is involved for each treatment; and
(6)   an assessment by the patient and physician together as to what treatments may be viable for curing the particular illness.

Each of these factors requires a detailed disclosure of information by the physician. This is especially so for the sixth factor since assessment involves a ranking of the treatments which presupposes that the patient has understood and retained all the medical treatments disclosed. Understanding this information involves a complex psychological process, which takes a substantial amount of time to achieve. The more accurately and effectively a physician explicates the treatments, the more completely a patient will understand the information disclosed. This further ensures that the patient, given his/her level of education and reflectiveness, will retain more information and thereby give a substantially informed consent based on a substantial understanding of the procedures involved in the treatments. Nothing less than this can be considered sufficient for an informed consent on the autonomy-enhancing model since the patient would lack sufficient detail of the treatments, and an informed consent could not be given.

The four important conditions for substantial understanding are minimally:

1.   Open communication;
2.   Shared understanding;
3.   Relevancy of information disclosed; and
4.   Sparing use of medical jargon by physician.

It should be noted that these four conditions do not exhaust all the conditions necessary for a patient to substantially understand the medical treatments.

(1) *Open communication* has several important requirements: (1) honest communication of all the relevant medical treatments and their risks and benefits; (2) the development of trust and respect between physician and patient; (3) communication without pretension or the use of other manipulators that inhibit genuine communication; and (4) an empathetic attitude on the part of the physician towards the patient – i.e., the physician must, in effect, put himself/herself in the patient's medical situation to determine how to disclose information about the treatments as clearly as possible to ensure understanding. A patient's illness has many subjective features which shapes his/her whole experience as a person. In other words, since a patient's whole person is affected by an illness, s(he) must be cured as a whole person despite his/her personal/subjective idiosyncrasies and intricacies.

I will only briefly focus on communication here since I will subsequently devote one chapter to the intricacies and complexities of the physician-patient relationship[2] and effective communication.[3] Generally, communication may be characterized as an exchange between two individuals that has (in this case) the overriding purpose of giving information and assisting understanding. The initial exchange is crucially important since it immediately establishes the character and quality of the physician-patient relationship. First impressions are important; if there is immediate friction or hostility between physician-patient, a relationship of open, honest communication can never be developed. Communication will only take place through psychological manipulators and effective communication will never occur. Most human relationships are formed on the basis of an immediate, intuitive judgment that turns out to be quite accurate on further reflection.

The most serious consequences of a fundamental lack of communication is that the trust and honesty that is necessary between physician and patient can never be achieved. Further, the patient will not be able to give an informed consent because of the lack of trust and confidence that the physician will, in fact, disclose all the information that is relevant to the patient. The physician will never have adequate knowledge about the patient due to his/her hostility and therefore will be unable to adequately disclose the relevant treatments that are required for an informed consent. The obvious solution to such a challenge is to seek the counsel of another physician who is more amenable to the needs of the patient. The physician-patient relationship is crucially important to develop and nurture, and should not be undermined, at the outset, by the incompatibilities of two individuals.

(2) *Shared Understanding.* Effective, unbiased and non-manipulative communication between physician and patient is important for a shared understanding of the patient's illness since it is necessary for the physician to disclose all the medical treatments available to the patient. Shared understanding occurs when both the physician and the patient understands the details of the patient's personal values, goals, beliefs, and life plans. In addition, the patient must understand that the physician is a person who operates within certain medical constraints that are, in effect, beyond his/her control. This is part of the foundational element of a substantial understanding between patient and physician; each person must comprehend the other in a subjective, person-to-person manner, which allows each person to communicate with one another openly and honestly, without manipulation or possible disingenuousness. The patient's feelings of vulnerability due to illness can be greatly lessened with a shared understanding between physician and patient.

There is an important distinction between "shared understanding" and "ordinary understanding". Shared understanding is based on a reciprocal understanding between patient and physician, which is a central feature of a substantial understanding of the medical treatments. Ordinary understanding consists of the physician communicating only the facts of the treatments and their risks and benefits without attempting to take the patient's medical and personal values into consideration. It is not sufficient for the physician to simply communicate the facts of the treatments and the risks and benefits since the physician must "personalize" the treatments to the particular patient. The personal features of the patient and his/her illness must be determined through effective communication and a "shared" understanding between physician and patient.

(3) *Relevancy of information disclosed.* The physician must also determine which information is personally *relevant* to disclose about the medical treatments. Initially, the physician must disclose all the treatments available, and the patient and physician must eliminate the irrelevant treatments together, evaluating the remaining treatments in

greater detail. It should never be the physician's sole responsibility to decide which treatments are relevant to a particular patient. Relevancy is difficult to determine because it is relative to the cognitive and emotional states of the patient. The personal and psychological aspects of a patient are difficult to unravel without communicating with the patient. Ensuring that a patient is included in the process of choosing the treatments invites the patient into the decision-making process of how to cure his/her own illness. This, in turn, ensures that the patient feels more comfortable, more secure, less vulnerable and more in control of his/her treatment options. Shared decision making of this sort also ensures that the patient is competent to decide what treatment s(he) will undergo, and this usually results in faster recovery for patients.

(4) *Medical Jargon.* Another condition for achieving substantial understanding is for physicians to use medical terminology that could be easily understood by the patient. If the treatments are outlined by the physician in a technical manner, the patient will not understand the treatment. The physician should be aware that s(he) is immersed in medical jargon that has taken many years to master. When medical language becomes second nature to the physician, s(he) may unintentionally disclose the medical treatments in a technical manner. Physicians should remember that medical terminology is a convenient short-hand; but it can and must be communicated so that the average patient can understand the treatments. The patient has no medical training, and although patients are better informed about health matters today than say a decade or so ago, technical jargon can make it impossible for some patients to understand the details of treatment.

Thus, the physician should be careful about how s(he) describes the treatments available to the patient. This difficulty in communication is exacerbated if the patient does not speak English well or is illiterate. In such cases, the patient may be completely lost and a translator must be brought in or a medical professional well acquainted with the patient's language. The situation is especially problematic with patients who may speak English well enough, yet still not have a substantial understanding of the treatments disclosed. The patient may not want to appear completely ignorant, and s(he) may pretend to understand the procedures when in fact s(he) only understood small portions of the information disclosed. When information is disclosed in a language that is foreign to the patient, his/her retention will obviously be further reduced since s(he) will find the medical procedures too technical to understand. In such cases, the physician must take additional steps to ensure that the patient understands the medical treatments disclosed.

III. Possible Difficulties in Achieving Patient Understanding

A substantial understanding of the treatments is difficult to achieve for some patients. The degree of the difficulty in achieving a substantial understanding depends on many factors. Some of these difficulties in understanding are due to the following factors:

1. *Patients differ in levels of education*, which leads to differing levels of understanding and literacy;
2. Patients differ in their *capacities for reflectiveness*; and
3. *Psychological factors* may influence a patient's capacity for understanding. Some of these factors are: (i) fatigue; (ii) relentless pain; and (iii) feelings of hopelessness and depression.

1. *Differing levels of education* affect how, or even whether, a patient will grasp the treatments and the amount of time needed to assimilate the information. Patients with secondary and post-secondary education do not pose as serious a problem for physicians as patients who have no secondary education. The latter group of individuals make the practice of achieving substantial understanding of medical treatments especially difficult. These difficulties, however, are surmountable. The less education a patient has, the more clearly and simply must the treatments be explained by the physician. In addition, it may be essential for physicians to take extra time to disclose and repeat the treatments in order for the patient to achieve a "substantial" understanding. However, these drawbacks are not completely detrimental to the process of understanding involved in giving an informed consent. Patients with lower educational levels may need extra attention to understand the treatments; however, they should still be able to achieve

substantial understanding about treatments which can lead to an informed consent.

The most effective way for a physician to determine a patient's educational level is for the physician and patient to engage in honest and open communication. The important point to recognize is that the physician can intuitively make an educational assessment of the patient while communicating without being condescending, manipulative or authoritarian. Given open, honest communication some patients may even directly admit that they have difficulties understanding certain medical procedures, and that there is a need to have the information repeated to ensure that the patient has substantially understood the treatment(s). This need not be a negative judgment about how the physician disclosed the treatments; instead, it is valuable for the physician to ensure that the patient understands the treatments and can thereby give an informed consent.

2. *Differing levels of patient reflectiveness* may also affect a patient's understanding of the treatments. It is relatively simple for a physician to determine whether a patient is reflective so that s(he) will not make a hasty decision in favor of a medical treatment. Typically, reflective patients: (1) insist on having an adequate amount of time to think about the treatments, and how each treatment may affect the patient; (2) ask relevant questions about certain important aspects of medical treatments that they didn't initially understand; and (3) decide in favor of a medical treatment on the basis of his/her beliefs, values, goals and life plans.

Reflectiveness does not, in principle, depend on the patient's level of education. Most individuals are reflective at least minimally, although the quality and degree of a patient's reflective capacity may vary substantially. Some patients may be reflective enough to think about the treatments disclosed by the physician, but may decide in favor of a treatment hastily, not taking the time to reflect on the treatments and their possible side effects. Such patients usually fail to have a coherent set of values, goals and life plans to make an autonomous choice about a medical treatment. There are also some completely unreflective patients and they pose the most severe difficulties for the physician. In such a case, the physician must guide a patient's thinking in an unbiased manner such that s(he) could make a decision which is reflective enough, demonstrating that s(he) has in fact understood and reflected on the information disclosed by the physician. Because of the importance of reflective awareness in achieving substantial understanding and a rational decision, a major part of the next chapter will be devoted to these issues.

3. *Psychological factors influencing understanding.* There are also three psychological factors that may influence a patient's understanding of medical treatments:

(i)   Fatigue;
(ii) Relentless pain; and
(iii) Feelings of hopelessness and depression.

(i) *Fatigue* may have a substantial effect on the patient's ability to think, retain information, and rationally assess information. Fatigue may be caused by a patient's inability to relax or sleep due to physical and/or psychological hardships but it is often caused by the illness itself. More relay time and repetitions may be needed for such patients to fully understand the treatments disclosed by the physician owing to the negative effect that fatigue has on memory capacity. The patient may also need a good night sleep before s(he) could make a proper decision in favor of a treatment that is intended to be based on a substantial understanding. Fatigue may also cause confusion and anxiety in the patient making it more difficult for him/her to make a rational, reflective decision. Most physicians are aware of these psychological influences but they may suppress them because of time pressures and caring for a large number of patients.

(ii) *Relentless pain* could also affect a patient's capacity for understanding information about treatments since if a patient is in constant pain, s(he) may experience depression and feelings of vulnerability. All the patient usually desires is to have his/her pain and discomfort alleviated as soon as possible. Such patients will usually "frame" treatment solutions to their diseases hastily and unreflectively. Physicians, upon recognition of such difficulties, must then guide a patient's thinking processes in deriving a treatment that is consistent with his/her values, goals, and deeply held beliefs prior to the illness. In this way, the patient may be able to "step back" from his/her pain, or at least reflect on how it was before his/her illness, and make a decision that is based on substantial understanding of the treatments.

(iii) *Feelings of hopelessness and depression* may be detrimental to a patient's capacity for understanding because these feelings can irrationally sway an individual towards treatments s(he) would not otherwise choose. The time available for chronic patients to have a normal life is usually drastically shortened upon being diagnosed with the disease. This is especially relevant for chronic disease patients who discover that their lives will be shortened because of the illness. They will "frame" the treatments differently from a patient who has an acute illness and will be undergoing a routine procedure after which time the patient will recover and resume his/her normal activities within a few weeks. The chronic disease patient will typically "frame" his/her decision in a way that is biased towards death, hopelessness and futility. The physician must keep this in mind since a chronic patient's decision in favor of a treatment will usually be irrational, lack understanding and therefore not be informed. One possible solution may be for the physician to guide the patient's thinking in a way that best reflects the patient's values, goals and life plans prior to his/her illness, which presupposes that the physician has known the patient for a prolonged time.

IV. Tests for Patient Understanding

There are several practical tests a physician could use to determine whether a patient really understands the treatments and their risks and benefits. First, the physician can ask the patient to repeat the treatments in his/her own words. In the process, the physician will be able to determine if the patient actually understood the treatments. This repetition focuses on the memory capability of the patient. There are some alarming statistics about the patient's retention of information in medical situations. In one report, 30 percent of patients were unable to say why the medical procedure was to be performed, while 43 percent of patients were unable to recall even one of the risks of the medical treatments only a short time after the information was disclosed.[4] These results force physicians to find ways of maximizing patient understanding when several detailed treatments are outlined.

A second way to ensure that patients understand the treatments is for the physician to disclose the information over several sessions instead of one long session, while asking the patient after each session to explain the treatment(s) disclosed during that session and/or the previous session (if there was one). After the last session, the patient must explain all the treatments disclosed by the physician. This gives the physician a good idea whether the patient understood the treatments. The more successfully (i.e., with as few errors as possible) a patient repeats all the treatments outlined, the more substantially the patient understood the information outlined by the physician. These step-by-step explanations serve to reinforce the treatments for the patient so that s(he) does not merely recall them, but will in the process know quite a bit more about the details of the treatments. This strategy seems to promise a better success rate, owing to the constant reinforcement of the information than the first test, which only stresses that a patient accurately repeat the information after all the disclosure of treatments.

By using these two strategies, physicians can ensure that their patients have substantially understood all the treatments. This is important because without a substantial understanding of the medical procedures, patients cannot possibly make an autonomous and rational decision about their treatment, and an informed consent cannot be achieved. Since physicians have a moral, if not a legal, duty to ensure that patients give an informed consent, they also have a duty to ensure that their patients have a substantial understanding of the treatments. These two tests adequately determine a patient's capacity for understanding. If the patient fails any one of these tests, the physician must repeat the process until the tests are passed.

Making autonomous, substantially understood decisions must be an important precondition for making rationally informed decisions, an issue to be examined in detail in the next chapter. One fundamental stumbling block in making rational decisions is that some patients make decisions in favor of a medical treatment on the basis of partly informed medical treatments. Such gaps in information are usually filled inaccurately and irrationally by the patient in order to give consent for a medical treatment. The physician must ensure that the patient has a substantial understanding of all the details of the treatments and their risks and benefits. Only in this way can an informed consent be achieved.

Notes

1. A visual representation of these facts is presented in Figure 4.1 below.
2. Chapter 6 will focus on how to develop an effective physician-patient relationship.
3. Chapter 7 will concentrate on effective communication as an important condition for developing an effective physician-patient relationship in which open trust and honesty are fostered.
4. These statistics are from "Informed Consent: Pondering a New Piece of the Puzzle". *Journal of Clinical Ethics*, fall, 1994, p.245.

Chapter 5

Rational Decision Making
In Informed Consent

The third condition for achieving informed consent is rational decision making. This is probably the most complex aspect of achieving an informed consent since it involves many idiosyncratic subjective and objective factors. If the patient's decision does not square with the paradigm of rational deliberation, an autonomous decision cannot be achieved by the patient. The physician must therefore take appropriate steps to ensure that the patient makes a rational decision about his/her medical treatments. A rational decision may be defined as

> a decision that is consistent with a patient's values, goals, beliefs and life plans, which isn't irrationally influenced by biases and prejudices that are irrelevant to the decision being made.

There are two common reasons why patients make irrational decisions:

(1) The psychological effects of medication or prolonged pain; and
(2) A lack of coherence among the patient's beliefs, values and life plans.

The first difficulty can be overcome through patience and diligence on the part of the physician and patient. The second difficulty is quite a bit more difficult to resolve.

(1) If a patient is on medication, it may hinder a patient's ability to achieve rational thinking. In such a case, the physician should either advise that the patient stop taking the specific medications for twelve, twenty four or even forty eight hours prior to a making decision in favor of a treatment, and/or guide the patient in his/her decision making processes. This last feature is more complex than is apparent on the surface because sometimes a physician may guide the patient's decision by unintentionally projecting some of his/her values, outcomes and conclusions onto the patient in a way that may seem paternalistic. On the autonomy-enhancing model, any paternalistic decision making is not permissible since it violates a patient's capacity for making rational decisions, and therefore autonomous decisions. Physicians must therefore ensure that they are *guiding* the patient but not prescribing what they consider to be the most beneficial treatments. To 'guide' means to 'think along with' the patient, helping the patient to deliberate rationally and reflectively. This process is typically most effective when physicians keep asking the patient relevant questions about the treatment(s) available in order to ensure that the patient has, in fact, understood them.

(2) Chronic care patients who experience continuous pain over a prolonged period of time and who have been prescribed mind debilitating medication are not uncommon in medical settings; it is for this reason that the physicians must develop special procedures to ensure the patient makes a proper decision in favor of a treatment. It is obvious, however, that physicians cannot always ensure that a rational decision is made by each patient; however, if a patient has substantial self-knowledge as to his/her deeply held values and beliefs, then an informed consent could will ultimately be achieved. In other words, the patient must have a coherent sense of self in order to be able to make important decisions about his/her health. If a patient lacks a coherent sense of self, s(he) will instinctively and hastily make decisions that may be influenced by factors that are irrelevant to the decision. For such individuals, making the right decision in favor of a medical treatment is a matter of luck, and a rational, reflective decision is difficult to achieve owing to the hastiness of the decision. Unreflective individuals cannot give an adequately informed consent for a medical intervention.[1]

It is difficult to estimate what percentage of patients lack the self-knowledge required to know their values and beliefs. We are supposedly the most reflective and informed culture in history, being sometimes referred to as the "autonomy culture". Medical information is available to every person that has access to television learning channels, radio, computer internet, or a public library. However, despite such preponderance of medical information and its ease of access, many individuals still remain ignorant about medical procedures. Thus, such patients find it difficult to make an informed and rational decision in favor of a medical treatment. Such reported observations, however, mostly concern epistemological facts about human beings, issues that are not directly the primary focus of this study. It is therefore necessary to exclude from consideration some of the inherent difficulties that unreflective patients pose to the process of achieving an informed consent.

There is another reason why patients who lack self-knowledge are excluded from the present study. It is difficult and controversial enough to state the conditions of a rational informed consent for those patients who have a consistent set of beliefs and values. Illness alone usually substantially influences a patient's judgments and capacity for rational assessment. If the physician has been familiar with the patient for a long time, the physician may be aware when the patient is making an irrational decision, or a decision that is out of character. It is only at this stage in the maturity of the physician-patient relationship that the physician could 'guide' a patient's thinking to ensure that the patient makes a rational decision in favor of a treatment. For unreflective patients, the problem of achieving an informed consent is multiplied many times. This is shown in Figure 5.1. The patients who lack an adequately coherent set of beliefs cannot make rational and autonomous decisions due to their lack of self knowledge. This is reflected in the last bar at the right and the right side of the middle bar in Figure 5.1.

Figure 5.1

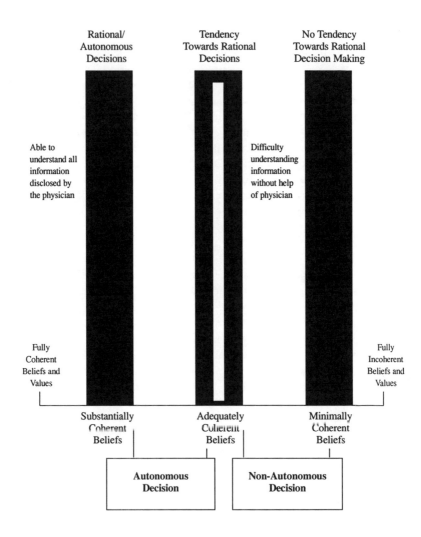

Rational/
Autonomous
Decisions

Tendency
Towards Rational
Decisions

No Tendency
Towards Rational
Decision Making

Able to
understand all
information
disclosed by
the physician

Difficulty
understanding
information
without help
of physician

Fully
Coherent
Beliefs and
Values

Fully
Incoherent
Beliefs and
Values

Substantially
Coherent
Beliefs

Adequately
Coherent
Beliefs

Minimally
Coherent
Beliefs

Autonomous
Decision

Non-Autonomous
Decision

There are subjective and objective dimensions of rational decision making that physicians need to take account. The subjective dimensions of rational decision making consist of the patient's beliefs and values which takes a substantial amount of time for the physician to become aware of for each patient. The objective dimensions of rational decision making are facilitated through effective communication and an effective physician-patient relationship.

I. The subjective dimensions consist of:
    (1)   self-knowledge;
    (2)   moral self-development;
    (3)   deliberation;
    (4)   erroneous or mistaken cognitive processes underlying decision making; and
    (5)   reflective awareness.

II. The objective dimensions consist of:
    (1)   shared decision making between physician and patient; and
    (2)   making decisions that are free from manipulative influences.

Both the subjective and objective dimensions are necessary for rational decision making and these conditions must be satisfied to achieve a rational decision in favor of a treatment. However, the subjective, personal dimensions of rational decision making are fundamental to making an autonomous decision, since without the objective features an autonomous decision cannot be achieved. The subjective features listed above will be examined in this chapter, while the objective features will be examined in the next chapter.

I. Subjective Dimensions of Rational Decision Making

(1) Self-knowledge may be defined as an individual's awareness of his/her beliefs as forming a unified character that is consistent over time. Every reflective person strives to ensure that s(he) has a coherent sense of self that has unchanging beliefs, values and goals forming

his/her life plans. These beliefs and values create the patient's sense of personhood, providing what is important for his/her sense of well being. For most reflective individuals, the process of self-understanding is a constant preoccupation throughout their lives. When an individual has self-knowledge, s(he) is usually able to predict his/her responses and decisions, and thereby also know what actions to take in order to preserve his/her beliefs and to keep them consistent. Any action or decision that fails this consistency criterion is not rational, and ought not to be pursued. Actions and decisions that are, in principle, autonomous should be rational and consistent; such actions must cohere with those aspects that make up the permanent self. Each individual can become aware of these personal and permanent aspects of the self through self-observation or introspection. There are three main features of self-knowledge:

(i) *An awareness of character traits.* Through introspection and self-analysis, an individual must be able determine whether s(he) is kind, gentle, generous, sympathetic, honest, forthright, virtuous or devious, rough, unmotivated, egoistical, dishonest, evil or a combination of these extremes. Most reflective individuals may be characterized as being somewhere between these extremes. We gain such knowledge by being reflective about our past actions and noticing patterns of action over time. Most individuals tend to act consistently over time and could make observations about themselves on that basis. An accumulation of such observations about ourselves results in a substantial knowledge of our values, goals and beliefs. This self-knowledge will facilitate the process of making informed medical decisions that may affect a patient's life.

(ii) *An awareness of belief structures.* Beliefs may be distinguished into different systems of belief such as religious, moral, epistemological, and psychological. Most self-reflective individuals can become aware of their belief structures through introspection and observing their actions. Our belief systems form networks of beliefs and act as foundations for other beliefs. There are few systems of beliefs, and many network beliefs. The more reflective an individual is, the more precise will be her/his awareness of such beliefs. A recognition of the networks that are operational in our belief structures may be helpful in determining our subsidiary beliefs; and this, in turn, gives us the self-knowledge to make decisions in favor of a treatment.

(iii) *A recognition of belief coherence or consistency.* Coherence or consistency are closely related features of each individual's belief structures. An individual has a consistent set of beliefs if s(he) has rejected contradictory beliefs from her/his system of beliefs, so that s(he) can act on the basis of a consistent set of principles. A coherent system of beliefs is the product of removing inconsistency from one's system-beliefs. Consistency is a necessary condition for coherence but it may not be necessary and sufficient. Coherence and consistency work together in forming a system-belief that is reliable and permanent. An individual must become aware of his/her own systems and networks of belief before s(he) can become aware of whether the beliefs are coherent and consistent. For instance, if an individual knows that s(he) is an honest person and is consistently guided by the principle of honesty, then even if a situation should arise in which lying is a temptation, s(he) must suppress the urge to go against his/her system-beliefs.

Autonomous individuals possess a well-developed and immediate knowledge of their permanent self consisting of their system-beliefs and character traits. Such information is distinctive of the particular person and cannot be known without self-knowledge, and this involves a long complicated process that takes a substantial amount of time to develop. This information must be communicated by the patient to the physician who needs to be aware of some of these subjective aspects in order to help patients achieve a rational and informed consent. If a physician has a recognition of a patient's beliefs, values and character traits, s(he) will be able to determine much more easily what information the patient needs to make an autonomous decision in favor of a medical treatment, since the physician will be able to give the most important and relevant information to the patient. Needless to say, the patient must have self-knowledge before s(he) could communicate his/her beliefs, values and life plans to the physician. When a patient has the required degree of self-knowledge, the task of giving a properly informed consent is facilitated for both the patient and the physician. The physician doesn't need to second-guess the patient's wishes in case of medical difficulties. Consider the following medical situation:

> A 50-year-old woman was diagnosed as having acute myeloid leukaemia, and in spite of the treatment was dying in the hospital. The physician has known the patient for years. She has told the physician in no uncertain terms that if she got seriously ill she wanted to know everything about her illness, even if it was fatal, since she is strongly committed to the principle of honesty. When the woman inquired, the physician disclosed the exact diagnosis.

In this situation, there was no dilemma for the physician -- the physician knew what the patient wanted to know based on her express instructions to the physician prior to the procedure which was derived on the basis of an autonomous, rational understanding and the physician simply disclosed the information without second-guessing or being concerned whether the negative diagnosis could lead to depression. If the patient informed the physician that she could not tolerate bad news and was sometimes unable to cope with it, the physician may have considered it better not to disclose the information. However, this is to fail to inform the patient of important information she may need in order to make further decisions about her health. The physician should therefore find some way to disclose the information as sensitively as possible.

(2) *Moral Self-Development*. Another important dimension of rational decision making requires that the patient must have a developed or mature moral self. A moral self can be defined as

a self that is aware of and consistently adheres to certain *prima facie* moral principles, these moral principles becoming guidelines for consistent action and moral decision making.

Developing a moral self takes a substantial amount of self-discipline and any decisions or actions that fail to cohere with an individual's moral principles must be considered irrational, and must therefore be rejected. Some individuals may feel tempted to act on inconsistent principles; especially if they feel vulnerable, as when a patient is ill. However, such actions are not only irrational but non-autonomous since the person has suppressed his/her moral principles in favor of an irrational impulse that led him/her to act in a way that was typically contradictory to his/her deeply held principles. The moral self that was once in complete control is now weakened by the patient's bodily discomforts and psychological stresses. Mercifully, not all patients fall into this difficulty. Consider the following medical situation:

A 44 year-old premenopausal woman has recently discovered a breast mass. Surgery was an alternative that she chose as a quick way of fixing the medical problem. Before surgery, the woman explicitly told the physician that if anything unusual was found during surgery that this was disclosed to her. She says: "I want to know everything about my body, regardless of whether it is good or bad". The physician has known the patient for about two years and is aware that she adheres to the moral principle of truth-telling, and that she is kind, self-disciplined, courageous and usually a rational decision maker who makes autonomous decisions.

The woman undergoes surgery during which time a 3.5-cm ductal carcinoma with no lymph node involvement that is estrogen receptor positive is detected. Chest roentgenogram, bone scan, and liver function tests reveal no evidence of metastasis. The patient was recently divorced and has gone back to work as a research assistant to support herself. What should the physician say to the patient?

Since the patient gave the physician express instructions prior to the procedure to disclose any new developments about her disease and the health conditions of her body, the physician has a moral duty to disclose the negative facts about her health. The woman seems to have an adequate amount of self-knowledge to clearly express her intentions to the physician and, it may be assumed that she has a well-developed reflective moral self. The patient has a basic right to know about the condition of her body in all medical situations. The information about the carcinoma may have to be disclosed sensitively and sympathetically by the physician; however, the important point is that if a physician knows the patient well enough, or express instructions are given to the physician based on a mature self-knowledge (as in this case), there is no real dilemma for the physician as to whether or not to disclose the nature of the medical condition. To respect a patient's autonomy and moral self, the physician must disclose the information about her health.

The situation may have been different if: (1) the woman did not clearly tell the physician that she wants to know everything about her medical situation; and (2) the physician has only known the patient for a few weeks, and had little time to communicate with her. Even if a patient has already endured enough medical hardships, and she has not stated that she wants to know everything about her condition, she still has a right to know everything; however, telling the patient at this particular time still might be devastating to her. It then follows that the physician may decide not to disclose the information to the woman. This view is more in accord with the harm-avoidance model of informed consent which asserts that patients must be spared from harm even if that means undermining a patient's autonomy. This view is unacceptable since it suggests a type of physician-authoritarianism and paternalism both of which typically leads to an uninformed consent. Other physicians might still feel compelled to disclose the information in the most sensitive and caring way possible, although the news may be painful to the woman. On the autonomy-enhancing model developed here, the physician must always respect a patient's autonomy, and not disclosing important information about the patient's medical condition undermines the patient's basic right to know what is happening to her body, and this can be considered a kind of paternalistic manipulation. Thus, the physician has a duty to first and foremost disclose all the information to the patient.

(3) *Deliberation.* Deliberation is generally characterized as a mental process directed towards some object or state of affairs with a view to reaching a decision to act. There are three stages of effective deliberation:

(i) *First order thinking* about the facts of the medical treatment as presented by the physician;
(ii) An *evaluation* by the patient and physician as to which medical facts are especially relevant for the patient and how the treatment will affect the patient; and
(iii) *Reflective deliberation* or second order deliberation is a test of whether the patient's initial assessment of the medical procedure was correct and not based on biases, prejudices, or other irrational procedures.

The patient must ensure that s(he) has effectively "framed" the treatment s(he) has decided on. At the second stage of deliberation, the patient formulates a personalized interpretation of the treatments available to the patient. The success of this process depends on how thoroughly the patient has deliberated on the exact details of the information presented, and how well the patient has kept all irrational impulses to a minimum.

(i) *First order thinking* is characterized for the purposes of decision-making as an active process of thinking directed towards some object or situation with a view to reaching a rational and autonomous decision. This characterization involves an active consideration of the facts by the patient of the treatments involved. This is a first order process since there is no further consideration needed except the facts of the various treatments as initially outlined by the physician. By prolonging the first stage of deliberation as long as possible, the patient will more clearly understand and deliberate on all the risks and benefits of the treatments, and thus make an adequate decision in favor of a treatment. Part of the initial deliberation may focus on how the particular treatments will influence the patient's life, and for how long. These facts are important for the evaluative stage of the deliberative process.

(ii) *The evaluative stage of deliberation* involves assessing the various treatments and weighing the benefits and risks of each treatment. This stage of deliberation focuses on assessment. It is a process of eliminating the irrelevant treatments by deliberating about each one and ultimately producing three or four realistic treatment options that can be further evaluated.[2] At this stage, the information that is disclosed by the physician must be thorough; all medical terms must be clearly explained and the possible (even if remote) complications must be outlined, for evaluation by the patient. The patient must ultimately choose the treatment that best suits his/her medical situation and life, such as his/her career, family, or interests.

The patient must also evaluate the information about the treatment options chosen on the basis of his/her deeply held beliefs, values, goals and life plans. It is crucial at this stage for the patient to have a coherent set of beliefs and values from which to evaluate the medical procedures. Without a "substantially" coherent set of foundational beliefs, the patient may have additional difficulties in deciding in favor of treatments. In such a case, the process of deliberation will take substantially longer to achieve; however, it is the physician's duty to ensure that the patient makes an autonomous decision that is consistent with his/her beliefs and values, even if they are not completely coherent. Such individuals will fall under the category of moderately reflective in Figure 5.2 below, and only have a 50 to 70 percent chance of making an autonomous decision.

The really difficult cases concern patients that are unable to deliberate much beyond the facts of the medical treatments outlined. Such individuals seem to have no recognition or access to their deeply held values and beliefs. Individuals who fall below the 50 percent category in Figure 5.2 are unable to determine their belief-structures nor which values will effect their decisions. To deal with the issues of how

Figure 5.2

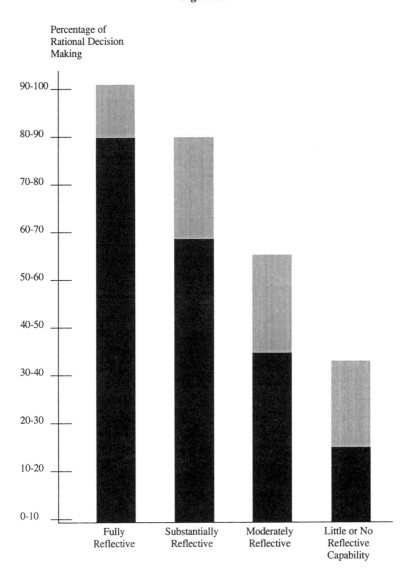

Percentage of
Rational Decision
Making

a medical practitioner would go about ensuring that such patients at least make adequately rational decisions in favor of a treatment goes beyond the scope of this study. The main concern is with a sliding scale of individual reflectivity which starts with a minimally coherent set of beliefs (50-60% capacity for rational decision making), and, ends with a maximally reflective attitude and a consistent set of beliefs and values (60-80% capacity for rational decision making).

(iii) *Reflective Deliberation.* The successful achievement of reflective deliberation presupposes that the patient has evaluated his/her choice of treatments rationally, i.e., in a way that didn't involve any irrational emotional and/or psychological influences. This is a difficult stage of the deliberative process since in times of illness the patient feels is vulnerable due to pain and other kinds of distress. There are ways that physicians can help patients to be more reflective by ensuring that any possible errors in judgment do not occur. This is one of the tasks of the physician since without proper reflection the patient may fail to give an informed consent.

(4) *Erroneous Cognitive Processes Underlying Decision Making*

Errors in reasoning and judgment are not unusual when patients make decisions in favor of certain medical treatments due to the inherent vulnerabilities in (and created by) the medical setting.[3] These errors of reasoning and judgment are responsible for some patients' inability to make a rational decision in favor of a medical treatment. Erroneous beliefs may have a significant role in decision making since biased reasoning may arise while representing the information initially disclosed by the physician. Thus, the manner in which the patient interprets and internally represents the medical treatments is crucially important. There are two possible errors of judgment under uncertainty: (i) belief bias effects; and (ii) framing effects.

(i) *Belief Bias Effects.* A "bias" may be defined as a systematic tendency to emphasize factors that are peripheral or irrelevant to the decision being made or to ignore factors that are strictly relevant. In order for a patient to capture the cognitive processes underlying decision making, s(he) must become aware of the

"biases" which may be consciously or unconsciously utilized when making decisions. For Tversky and Kahneman, "belief bias effects" are defined as biases in "processing probability information". "Probability information" is roughly that which is needed for risk assessment.
In order to make a decision in favor of a medical treatment, patients must reach judgments about the probability of certain outcomes. This *perceived* probability of outcomes is crucial for making an informed decision about a medical treatment. Research has been conducted to ascertain the processes that are involved in making decisions about probabilities. Kahneman and Tversky proposed two heuristics, namely, (a) representativeness; and (b) availability, which can be used by patients in making decisions about medical probabilities.

(a) *Representativeness.* The "representative heuristic" influences and substantially biases a patient's decisions in ways that are unacceptable to autonomous decision making. The representativeness heuristic results in a decision that is biased by previous decisions that are representative of the decision at hand. For instance, if the patient has undergone a previous medical treatment, which was unsuccessful or painful, his/her decision may be influenced by that negative experiences and therefore (s)he will expect the previous treatment to be representative of the second one. Thus, the patient may erroneously decide against a medical treatment believing that it will be representative of the previous ones that failed, when in fact, this treatment may be successful in alleviating some, or all, of the medical discomfort that (s)he is experiencing. In this way, the patient may be led to errors and biases in reasoning when (s)he, either consciously or unconsciously, has internally represented the medical treatment in a biased manner.
(b) *Availability.* According to Tversky and Kahneman, patients may also make decisions based on the probability

associated with certain events that can be readily brought to mind. Probabilities that occur frequently are recalled quicker and applied to the situation at hand, even if they are not strictly relevant to it. However, most of us are aware of the fact that, just because a certain event can be called to mind with greater ease that doesn't necessarily make it the basis for an accurate decision. In fact, if a patient decides in favor of a given medical treatment too hastily without rationally considering all the risks and benefits, (s)he may indeed be influenced by the availability heuristic since his/her decision was derived, not from careful evaluations and assessments of the information presented, but from an intuition that was immediately grasped without rational calculation. This may lead to irrational decision making.

(ii)   *Framing Effects* are characterized as the way in which information is presented by the physician and interpreted by the patient. Patients may formulate a *personalized* representation of the treatments and, because of the way they are framed, may misinterpret the details of the treatments to fit their own framing projections and preferences, i.e., their own beliefs about the treatments but not the exact details of the treatments as disclosed by the physician. There are times when the patient may be faced with high risk prospects in his/her treatment. If the physician communicates this high risk directly in his/her disclosure of the treatment, then the patient may 'frame' the medical procedures solely in terms of risks rather than benefits or, alternatively, only in terms of successes rather than risks. For instance, if a patient perceives the options of surgery in terms of the probabilities of survival, this kind of "framing" may hinder the patient from simultaneously being able to perceive or understand the risk of death during surgery.

There are two ways patients unconsciously deal with risky information. First, the patient may be in a state of denial about the severity of his/her illness and may engage in wishful thinking which is self-deceptive and interferes with autonomous decision-making. For instance, a survival "frame" may prevent a patient from grasping that there may be a risk of death during surgery, and if this medical information is relevant in order for the patient to give properly informed permission to undergo a particular medical treatment, then the patient's choice of surgery is biased, making the decision nonautonomous. This kind of wishful thinking is usually engaged by patients who are chronically ill. Every patient, prior to getting ill, has the ultimate hope that (s)he will live for quite a long time. Yet when serious illness threatens an individual's life, his/her sense of integrity and personhood may be undermined, and (s)he will find it difficult to make a rational choice if s(he) is not reflective, disciplined and resolute about the medical situation and the treatments available.

Second, the patient may process the risk or inevitability of death due to illness by "framing" the treatments available in terms of risks of uncertainty. When dealing with risky treatment such as a bone-marrow transplantation or chemotherapy, the choices available to the patient may both have negative and uncertain results. The patient may have to make a decision between (1) prolonging his/her life by undergoing surgery, and perhaps prolonging pain and misery; or (2) not engaging in any medical procedures except pain killers, and accept death as a real option. Is it rational for cancer patients to refuse treatment? This is a difficult question to answer objectively because it depends on an individual's preferences and rationally calculated judgments. The final decision depends on the patient's beliefs and values. If a patient strongly believes in the sanctity of life, (s)he may opt for undergoing surgery and prolonging life, despite some of the later difficulties. However, if the patient believes in dying with dignity, (s)he may opt for minimizing the time (s)he must suffer with pain and uncertainty. As long as the patient's decision is consistent with his/her values, beliefs, and goals, and is not based on irrational impulse or fear, the patient has a right to decide whether or not to endure treatment.

II. Objective Dimensions of Rational Decision Making

There are two objective ways that the physician could ensure that patients make rational decisions and achieve a substantially autonomous decision: (1) shared decision making; and (2) ensuring that patients avoid misinterpretations arising from manipulative influences that result in an irrational decision.

These two objective features of rational decision making will be considered in detail in the next chapter as they are important and complex components of a trusting and effective physician-patient relationship. For the present, it is necessary to discuss reflective awareness, which is a second-order deliberation of the initial evaluation of the medical treatments. If reflective awareness is effective and successful, the patient can circumvent some of the irrational interpretations about the medical treatments outlined, and help to eliminate some of the belief-bias effects and framing effects in their decision making by stepping back from the initial decision and reassessing their judgment.

(5) *Reflective Awareness* is a process through which the mind becomes aware of its own operations. A more practical characterization is that reflective awareness is a process of examining our thinking processes, trying, for example, to determine how we derived our initial judgments and assessments. This is achieved by becoming introspective about our own thinking processes in order to retrace our initial deliberations. The terms 'introspective', 'reflective' and 'deliberative' have distinctive meanings and should not be conflated or considered to mean more or less the same process. Deliberative processes consist of our first-order, ordinary pre-reflective thinking, which has been examined above. In introspection, an individual must become aware of his/her own thinking processes that make up his/her first-order processes. Introspection is a process that makes it possible to be aware of ordinary, first-order deliberation and second order, reflective awareness. The evaluative stage of the awareness occurs at the reflective, second-order stage when the individual makes a judgment about his/her thinking processes. In other words, there is a level distinction between ordinary, first order awareness and reflection, which is assessment and evaluation of one's thinking processes.

Thus, reflective awareness is a second-order deliberative process, which requires that the patient evaluates his/her initial decisions in favor of a medical treatment. The process of reflective awareness is somewhat difficult to understand as it is usually described using phenomenological terminology. Reflective awareness is generally defined as a type of conscious, second-order reflection, and some individuals may have difficulty to adequately incorporate it into their decision-making methods. Some individuals may find it difficult to grasp the meaning of what constitutes second-order reflection, which is a form of introspection or 'turning back' on our initial interpretations and judgments. This state of mind or attitude is quite distinct from our ordinary, everyday pre-reflective deliberative processes, which is the foundation for reflective awareness.

Let me dwell a bit longer on the concept of introspection since it is a necessary condition for reflective awareness. Introspection requires memory and the imagination, and may be characterized as an active, intentional process of examining our beliefs and values, or any information that needs to be assessed at the reflective stage. This active stage of introspection is awareness understood as selective attention, as opposed to Titchener's old fashioned version of introspection that supposed introspection to be a kind of passive observation of the mind. This view is now assumed to be quite mistaken given current trends in psychology and the philosophy of mind. Selective awareness is a method by which a person attends to the inner contents of his/her mind to make selective observations and assessments.

Reflective awareness depends on one's ability to introspect since reflective awareness presupposes a deeper, more intense acquaintance. This further presupposes a high degree of clarity of mind, and a coherent, well-formulated set of beliefs, values, goals and life plans from which an individual can introspect. This second-order deliberation is crucially important for medical decisions since it is a procedure in which the patient has the ability to suspend judgment in favor of a medical treatment until s(he) is certain that the treatment s(he) chooses is the most likely option. This suspension of judgment is a necessary feature of reflective awareness since it is part of a methodology that ensures that a patient's decision is based on well-reasoned, autonomous judgments about a medical treatment.

Reflection is beneficial in ensuring that a patient makes a rational decision in favor of a medical treatment since it presupposes that the patient critically evaluates all the medical treatments disclosed by the physician and makes a decision that is consistent with his/her values, beliefs and life goals. This process also ensures that the decision made is rational and autonomous. This evaluative analysis takes a considerable amount of time to achieve and depends on the patient. Different individuals have different capacities for second-order reflection, and not every person is equally reflective. In addition, since illness and medication weakens a patient's reflective capacities, illness may extend the process of reflection even longer.

Thus, reflective awareness signifies more than the freedom to choose between treatments. It requires that a patient makes a reflective choice that represents his/her deeply held beliefs and preferences, not those of a brief or fleeting duration, but to seek out those that are a permanent and stable part of his/her life and experience. Patients are more than a bundle of individual behaviors; they are capable of reflective awareness which ensures that their decisions will be carefully calculated and thus morally autonomous.

When reflective awareness is effective, the physician will not be subject to as much uncertainty in obtaining a rational decision in favor of a medical procedure. It will be possible for physicians to be more confident in determining whether the patient has understood the information disclosed, and whether his/her decision was influenced by other irrelevant considerations. The physician can do this by being attentive to the kinds of questions that the patient asks and the kind of clarifications that the patient believes are critical to his/her making a proper medical decision. Most patients will make decisions that are consistent with the type of individuals that they are, and if the physician is aware of this, s(he) will have added confidence in assessing whether his/her patient has made a rational and autonomous decision.

But what if the physician, while disclosing the medical information, recognizes that his/her patient lacks adequate rational, reflective deliberation and simply decides in favor of a particular treatment in an unreflective manner? Does the physician have a duty to probe further in order to enable his/her patient to comprehend all the medical treatments presented more reflectively? On the autonomy-enhancing model, reflective deliberation is a central moral requirement of rational decision making and of an informed consent, and the physician does therefore have a moral duty to ensure that a patient's decisions are autonomous and calculative in nature, provided that the patient has self-knowledge and is only temporarily debilitated by illness. The physician could help the patient further reflect by guiding and encouraging the patient's thinking processes to reflect as deeply as possible on the risks and benefits of the treatments to ensure that the patient's decision is rational and autonomous. Some physicians may argue that this places an unwarranted burden on the physician since it is not the physician's responsibility to ensure that a rational decision is made in favor of a treatment. Instead, it is the patient's prerogative to make certain that his/her decisions are autonomous and most patients are able to achieve this. But while this may be the case for more than half of all patients, some patients may need more guidance than others in order to make a rational and reflective.

In summary, physicians may need to spend a substantial amount of time guiding some of their patient's thinking processes in order for some patients to make a rational and autonomous decision in favor of a medical treatment. Some patients may lack the second-order reflective awareness that is necessary to make assessments about their initial decisions. The physician should not expect the patient to proceed on his or her own since, given their medical condition, they may lack proper second order reflection and the basis for risk assessment in order to make a rational decision. This requires that the physician and patient engage in effective communication in order to reach a rational decision in favor of a medical treatment together. Effective communication, in turn, requires that an effective physician-patient relationship is developed and nurtured. I turn to these issues in the next two chapters.

Notes

1 . Individuals who are incapable of engaging in a sufficient degree of reflection required for rational decisions will be excluded from this study. On the autonomy-enhancing model, the rationality that an informed consent demands as a necessary condition is beyond such individuals' emotional and intellectual capability. In short, patients who do not have a coherent picture of the self will find it very difficult to make autonomous, rational and informed decisions. It is not the responsibility of physicians to guide such patients into forming a coherent set of beliefs and values. This is definitely beyond the physician's call of duty and perhaps even beyond the call of a psychologist.

2 . The number of treatments derived is unimportant. It must only be a manageable number so that the patient does not reach cognitive-information overload.

3 . Kahneman and Tversky wrote several articles on 'biases' and 'heuristics'. Some of the more relevant ones for my purposes are: (1) Kahneman, Daniel, & Tversky, Amos. "Choices, Frames and Values". *American Psychologist*, 1984, Volume 39(4), 341-350. (2) Kahneman, Daniel & Tversky, Amos. "Judgment Under Uncertainty: Heuristics and Biases". *Science*, (1974) 125, 1124-1131. (3) Tversky, A., and Kahneman, D. "The Framing of Decisions and the Psychology of Choice". *Science*, 211, 453-458.

Chapter 6

Effective Patient-Physician Relationship

The three conditions for an informed consent outlined so far are impossible to bring about without an effective patient-physician relationship which is best achieved through effective communication. The more compatible, sympathetic, open, honest and trusting the relationship between the physician and patient is, the more effective will be their verbal exchanges. The more intrinsic or extrinsic tensions[1] between the physician and patient, the less effectively they will communicate, and the less likelihood will a rational decision be made in favor of a treatment. Thus, it is necessary for the patient and physician to develop a compatible and effective relationship to ensure that the process of achieving an informed consent will be successful. I devote the next chapter to the conditions of effective communication between physician and patient that are necessary to achieve an informed consent. This chapter will be devoted to an examination of the factors that constitute an effective physician-patient relationship.

To develop and nurture an effective physician-patient relationship, the physician must have an awareness of the patient's beliefs and values. The physician must become aware of his/her patient as a person and not merely as a diseased body that needs medical attention. Every patient will have different needs for information-disclosure depending on their personal idiosyncrasies, and unless the physician is aware of them, s(he) will be ineffective in disclosing the relevant information about the treatments to the patient. Specifically, if a physician is not aware of the patient's psychological, medical, epistemological and intellectual make-up, s(he) will be unable to adequately understand the patient and thus will be unable to effectively "personalize" the information about treatments.

However, the patient must also be cognizant of the physician's personality. For instance, if a physician has a habit of being hasty and impatient, it is possible that s(he) will be unable to convey all the relevant information about the treatments available to the patient due to his/her lack of patience. If the patient suspects that this is a predominant personality trait of the physician, the patient will have to ask the physician whether the treatments disclosed by the physician included all the relevant treatments. This may require the physician to reflect on whether all the treatments were indeed disclosed. Open and honest communication between physician and patient is difficult under such circumstances and does not encourage the patient's trust in the physician. The patient must trust that the physician has disclosed all the information about the treatments to the patient, and the physician must trust that the patient has understood and rationally assessed all of the relevant medical treatments in order to achieve an autonomously informed consent. This reciprocal relationship of trust is one of the building blocks for an effective physician-patient relationship which will be examined in more detail in the next chapter.

There are two centrally important features of an effective physician-patient relationship:

I. Non-manipulative communication between physician and patient; and
II. Shared decision making between patient and physician.

The unacceptable practice of using manipulative techniques to communicate the medical treatments to the patient will be considered first since shared decision making is impossible without honest, open and non-manipulative communication between patient and physician. A physician who makes use of manipulative techniques erodes any possibility of developing an effective physician-patient relationship.

1. Non-Manipulative Communication Between Physician and Patient

The exchange between physician and patient in the process of informed consent must be free from manipulative influences. Such irrational influences on the part of the physician can lead to orchestrated decisions that are not substantially informed and in most cases are non-autonomous. Rather, the treatments must be outlined objectively (i.e., free from psychological manipulations) and in such a way as to take into account the patient's beliefs, values and life goals. There are four kinds of manipulations that may be used by physicians:

(1) coercion;
(2) persuasion;
(3) prioritizing of information presented; and
(4) tone of voice.

(1) *Coercion* is defined as intentional influences that pose or exaggerate a credible threat of unwanted and avoidable harm, that is so influential that the patient cannot resist acting to avoid it. In such a case, the patient would be consenting to treatment that is not necessarily in his/her best interest, and hence the decision made would be non-autonomous. This occurs most notably when the physician is dogmatically convinced that the patient should undergo a given medical treatment without recognizing the patient's values, beliefs, life goals or his/her previous medical history. If the patient submits to the physician's coercions and accepts a particular treatment, s(he) will non-autonomously agree with the physician's recommendation, yet still accept it.

Few physicians, even of the traditional, paternalistic kind, now use coercive techniques due to peer pressure and the extreme irrational response that it tends to produce in the patient. Sometimes physicians may use coercion only as a last resort if they believe that the patient is making an irrational decision by refusing a necessary treatment. For instance, if a patient should undergo surgery and yet irrationally decides against it, the physician may coerce the patient by saying "if you don't have surgery, you will die". This usually is an exaggeration, but it is sometimes used to convince the patient to undergo surgery as the quickest and more secure treatment. However, even though the patient made an irrational decision against surgery based on previous biases, the physician should resist using coercive techniques to convince a patient to undergo surgery. Instead, the physician should guide the patient's thinking so that s(he) will make a more rational decision the second time the treatments are outlined. Some patients initially make an irrational decision in favor of a treatment; after the second or third repetition of the treatments, the patient becomes convinced that his/her previous decision ought to be "reframed" and reconsidered.

(2) *Persuasion* may be characterized as the successful attempt to convince a patient through appeals to reason, or the emotions, in favor of a treatment that the physician thinks that the patient should undergo in order to improve his/her health. When a patient's beliefs are manipulated by the physician, the patient is persuaded to undergo a medical treatment that is not in accordance with the moral autonomy and integrity of the patient. This is the most complex type of manipulation since it may be difficult for the patient to correctly determine whether s(he) is being persuasively influenced by the physician. Sometimes the physician may persuade the patient so subtlety that the patient will be unaware of being persuaded, and therefore, s(he) remains unreflectively aware of whether his/her decision was informed and autonomous or uninformed and non-autonomous.

(3) *Prioritizing of the Treatments.* The order in which the physician presents the treatments, such as claiming that there is a primary, secondary or tertiary treatment to cure a particular medical condition, may influence a patient's decision. Patients may sometimes be influenced by the ordering of the medical treatments outlined since they may believe that the treatments that the physician presents first must be the most beneficial (painless and relatively risk-free) treatment while the second or third treatment may have additional difficulties. The physician can manipulate the patient by presenting what s(he) believes to be the most viable treatment first, such that by the time the physician discloses the fourth or fifth treatment, the patient may have reached his/her cognitive saturation point and won't be able to either

remember what was previously disclosed or to ascertain its importance. Therefore, the patient would opt for the first, second or third treatment depending on which one s(he) remembers most clearly. A possible solution may be for the patient to simply ask whether there is any importance attached to the ordering of the treatments. This at least makes the physician aware that the patient is reflective enough to make finer discriminations. Another possible way to circumvent such manipulations would be for the patient to ask that the treatments be presented in written form so that s(he) could read them over several times. This ensures that the patient could study all the possible medical treatments available not just the ones that were outlined first.

(4) *Tone of Voice.* If a physician speaks in a loud tone of voice this may give the patient a feeling of uneasiness towards the treatment. In other cases, patients may interpret loud voices as being authoritative; the authority carries over to the treatment that is suggested by the physician which may result in a non-autonomous acceptance of a treatment. Soft voices, on the other hand, may connote acceptance, less risk, openness and sympathy. Patients interpret verbal cues in a variety of non-rational ways, depending on a patient's state of vulnerability. Tone of voice can be a powerful manipulative technique and physicians must be reflective about their tone of voice as they are outlining the treatments to the patient.

On the autonomy-enhancing model, it is never acceptable for physicians to use any manipulative techniques to convince patients to agree that a particular medical treatment is in their best interest since such attitudes undermine a patient's autonomy, and erodes the physician-patient relationship. In addition, such manipulative techniques reinforce the much outmoded paternalistic model of medicine in which the physician is viewed as an authority. No consent is needed on this model since the physician assumes that s(he) knows what is in the patient's best interest. Consent under the traditional model focused on harm-avoidance above all else, even if that meant undermining a patient's autonomy. Currently, on the autonomy-enhancing model, all consent given by a patient must be autonomous and autonomy-enhancing. Thus, it is never acceptable for the physician to undermine a patient's autonomy and basic right of giving an informed consent.

Many physicians unintentionally use manipulative techniques since they are an inherent part of the fabric of the traditional model of medicine. Some of the justifications commonly used by physician's for using manipulative techniques are:

(i)   physician time constraints;
(ii) deficiency in a patient's psychological competency;
(iii) a lack of physician patience to disclose all the treatments;
(iv) an assumption that the patient's is unable to understand medical terminology; and
(v)   biases caused by a physician's personal dislike of his/her patient or character clashes.

For these reasons, the physician may feel justified in deciding which treatment the patient should undergo and then coerce or manipulate the patient into agreeing with the treatment. However, each of these justifications undermine a patient's right to self-determination and autonomy. Thus, on the autonomy-enhancing model, such rationalizations must be avoided. Because they are so common, it is important to examine these justifications in some detail to understand why some physicians may still be using them.

   (i) *Time constraints.* It is always possible for physicians to make a case for being overworked and overstressed due to the everyday pressures and long hours of work that is a part of a physician's professional work. Physicians may feel pressured for a multitude of reasons, such as being overburdened by too many patients, an insufficient number of medical personnel, and long hours at the hospital and office. However, this is the reality of a physician's professional life, and s(he) must find a way to overcome such constraints by perhaps (i) hiring assistants; (ii) giving additional responsibilities to the nursing or hospital staff; or (iii) by refusing to accept additional responsibilities if it isn't absolutely necessary. It is never justified for a physician to undermine a patient's autonomy and basic right to make an autonomous decision due to time constraints, except in justified emergency situations. Thus, the time constraint justification must not be an obstacle if the patient is to develop an effective physician-patient relationship.

(ii) *Deficiency in a patient's psychological competency.*[2] Every patient has a different level of intellectual and emotional intelligence. The physician must be aware of the patient's educational level before disclosing the medical treatments. Most patients are psychologically competent to make their own decisions in favor of a medical treatment. For the few patients that are prone to such psychological challenges, they should again be *guided* by the physician into making an autonomous decision in favor of a medical treatment. Under no circumstances is it permissible or justifiable for the physician to be manipulative or coercive. The physician has a duty to ensure informed consent with every patient (even with the educationally and psychologically challenged) and to ensure that the patient's decision is rational, reflective and autonomous.

(iii) *Lack of physician patience.* Physicians must allot a sufficient amount of time to disclose *all* the relevant treatments, and the risks and benefits. The disclosure of the treatment options is typically a time-consuming process, but the physician has a moral duty to ensure that s(he) spends as much time as is required for a particular patient to understand the information relayed. The time required will vary from patient to patient. For some patients, the physician may need to schedule several sessions to disclose the treatment options. It is crucially important that a physician accurately determine how much time is necessary to outline the treatments for each patient, and then take the time needed to ensure that the patient understands them.

(iv) *A Patient's inability to understand medical terminology.* Some physicians believe they have expert knowledge that cannot be understood by the lay person. This is a faulty assumption since every profession has its own technical jargon that most lay persons can understand, given all the ways they could attain such information such as through learning channels on the television, and self-help medical books. All technical terms can be explained in simple non-technical language that can be understood by individuals outside the medical profession; in other words, any technical terms can be translated into non-technical language so that it can be easily understood by the lay person. Failure to do so may be construed as a form of manipulation since unless a patient understands the treatments, s(he) will be unable to make an autonomous decision in favor of a treatment.

(v) *Character clashes.* Personality clashes between physician and patient are not uncommon occurrences in medical situations, yet few medical professionals ever regard it as having a significant impact on the patient's medical well being. Character clashes occur when there is personal friction between physician and patient for unknown reasons. In such cases, the physician may feel that it is permissible to be rude and condescending to the patient, this being no doubt a backlash from the old traditional, paternalistic view of medicine in which the physician is considered to be an authority. According to this outdated view, the patient is treated as if s(he) is incapable of making his/her own medical decisions. However, since the early 1970's with the focus on patient autonomy, this kind of paternalistic behavior has become unacceptable. Since the stress on autonomy became a critical aspect of informed consent, and the patient's cooperation in the decision of choosing the treatment options became essential for an autonomous decision in favor of a medical treatment and an informed consent, the nature of the physician-patient relationship had to change substantially from the old traditional, paternalistic relationship to a relationship in which both the patient and physician formed a partnership. Given the current stress on partnership-based relationships between physician and patient, it is never permissible for the physician to be rude or condescending to the patient. If personality clashes are detected by the patient, s(he) must switch physicians and find one that is compatible.

II. Shared Decision Making

The second feature of an effective physician-patient relationship is shared decision which consists of:

(1) Acknowledging uncertainty;
(2) Shared authority;
(3) Mutual trust and respect; and
(3) Respecting a patient's autonomy.

(1) *Acknowledging Uncertainty.* The notion of "shared decision making" is difficult for some physicians to accept because of the paternalistic tradition that has been in effect in medicine for centuries. Traditionally, medicine has been viewed by the general public as a stable, reliable profession, with few uncertainties. When a patient needs medical attention, it is now common for him/her to believe that the science of medicine will almost certainly cure the patient's illness. There has been a concern by medical professionals that shared decision making between patient and physician may result in a disclosure of some of the known uncertainties that physicians are acutely aware of in the science of medicine. Some physicians may feel that if the patient becomes aware of these medical uncertainties they may feel even more vulnerable, and that they may lack the confidence that they need to take risks. The patient usually acts on the assumption that s(he) can completely trust the medical enterprise to cure any ailment; however, this assumption is in some cases mistaken. Disclosing medical uncertainties is an implicit way for physicians to tell the patient that medicine is an art that is not free from trial and error. Thus, medicine is more analogous to an art than to science. There are many diseases that still have no cure, such as AIDS, multiple sclerosis, and many kinds of cancers. In addition, there are many more diseases discovered everyday for which there is no known cure.

The unknown dimensions of certain diseases make medicine much more unpredictable and uncertain, and some physicians would prefer to keep this uncertainty hidden from their patients since they want to uphold their professionalism and the trust that patient's have in them. Physicians prefer that patients have complete confidence that their illness will be cured by the treatment. In other words, physicians want to keep their professional image intact, even if that means keeping some valuable information concealed about the uncertain results of certain medical treatments. This is problematic because it undermines a patient's autonomy by making it impossible for the patient to refuse treatment if the probabilities of being cured are uncertain. In addition, shared decision making is difficult to achieve unless the physician explicitly expresses such uncertainties to the patient. Thus, on the autonomy-enhancing model, the physician has a duty to disclose such uncertainties to the patient.

Shared decision making may sometimes involve the "tension of uncertainty"[3] which highlights the fact that physicians must not only disclose information about medical treatments but they must also communicate any uncertainties about a medical treatment. This involves giving the patient information about the probabilities of success and failure for a particular medical treatment. The track record of a treatment is valuable information when a patient is making a decision in favor of a treatment. Patients may still choose treatments that have low probabilities of success; however, they will be able to decide for themselves whether they will take the risk, and this involves making an autonomous decision.

(2) *Sharing Authority.* "Sharing authority" in decision making does not necessarily mean that physicians and patients must make a joint decision about a medical treatment, but instead the patient and physician must each corroborate a decision about a medical treatment that reflects the patient's values, goals, beliefs and life plans. In the process of communication, the physician must guide the patient into becoming aware of his/her deeply held beliefs, values and goals in a non-judgmental, non-biased and non-prejudicial manner. This will ensure that the patient will be capable of making an autonomous decision in favor of a medical treatment. The ultimate goal of shared decision making is that the physician ensures the patient makes a substantially autonomous decision in favor of a medical treatment. However, if the physician and patient does not form a partnership-type relationship in which each person equally contributes to the decision making process, an autonomous decision in favor of a medical treatment will be difficult if not impossible to achieve.

Shared decision making consists of a kind of mutual dependency relationship between patient and physician. The physician cannot disclose the information about medical treatments without the personal knowledge of the patient, and the patient cannot make a decision without an adequate disclosure of medical treatments. Both the patient and physician are considered to be an authority in different ways, in that the patient is an authority about his/her personal goals, values and beliefs, and the physician is an authority on medical knowledge and the possible medical treatments that are available to the patient. A properly informed consent consists of both the patient's self-knowledge, and the physician's medical knowledge. Thus, such shared authority is an essential feature of an effective physician-patient relationship.

The old, traditional paternalistic model of the physician as a prescriber of medications and treatments has been dethroned. It has become a physician's implicit responsibility to ensure and assist that the patient to make an autonomous, rational, reflective and well understood decision about his/her medical treatments. This involves encouraging patients to make autonomous decisions in favor of medical treatments that will affect their lives. It is the patient who must determine for him/herself what medical procedures s(he) will endure.

(3) *Mutual Trust and Respect.* In order for shared decision making to be achieved, the patient and physician must fundamentally trust each other. An effective physician-patent relationship is built on trust. Due to the vulnerabilities of the medical profession's uncertainties and the patient's illness, mutual trust is essential to foster a relationship where the two parties can achieve open, honest communication. Mutual trust has two dimensions, one for the physician and one for the patient. The patient must trust that the physician will disclose all the treatment options honestly and openly to ensure that the patient can reach a rational and reflective decision in favor of a medical treatment. The physician must, in turn, trust that the patient will understand and use all the information competently and make a rational and autonomous decision about treatment. When I say that the physician trusts the patient, I mean that s(he) trusts that the patient has reflected on all the treatment options and has adequately assessed their risks and benefits. This means that the patient has understood all the information relayed and that s(he) communicated any difficulties in understanding the details of the treatment to the physician in order that they may be rectified and an informed consent achieved. This trust may take the form of an intuition on the part of the physician about his/her patient. However, there is also an implicit trust by the patient that the physician has disclosed all the treatments. Typically, mutual trust develops slowly

between patient and physician; however, it is necessary for an effective relationship.

Mutual respect is also an essential condition for establishing an effective physician-patient relationship. It takes a substantial amount of time, effort and maturity to develop an effective relationship that is based on mutual trust and respect. Trust is built on more than actions alone; effective communication between physician and patient is also required in achieving and giving an informed consent. Trust that is developed between physician and patient requires much more than the mere trust that a patient has that his/her physician has the medical expertise to perform the treatment adequately. Physicians and patients should not hesitate to also share their uncertainties with one another.

However, trust and respect between patient and physician are not easily acquired virtues. Physicians must strive to give both a diseased body and a diseased person its proper importance and where conflicts arise; they must reconcile whether they will give preference for a diseased body or a diseased person. On the autonomy-enhancing model presented here, a diseased person must take precedence over a diseased body since the patient must make an autonomous decision and must decide for him/herself as to the most appropriate treatment to cure his/her body. There is no necessary boundary between the body and the person since whatever happens to the body always influences the person but it is the person who must deal with the illness. Thus, the physician must deal with both dimensions of the person, and this presupposes certain principles of moral behavior that respects the whole person.

(4) *Respecting Autonomy.* The physician must respect a patient's autonomy by cultivating an effective relationship in which the patient is given a sufficient amount of time and space to make his/her own decisions in favor of a medical treatment. On the traditional, paternalistic model, patients were regarded as vulnerable children instead of autonomous adults. Illness may weaken a patient's ability to make autonomous decisions; however, the important point is that it doesn't eradicate it altogether. A patient that is chronically ill and/or in discomfort can still make autonomous decisions, although as mentioned above, the process of decision making in favor of a medical treatment may take considerably longer. However, the physician must not

erroneously assume that the patient will be completely incapable of making an autonomous decision. There are times that a physician may impatiently 'frame' the patient as being incapable of autonomous decision making, and thus either use manipulative techniques, or paternalistically prescribe a treatment on behalf of the patient. Unless there is a good reason to assume that a patient lacks a sense of self and autonomy (i.e., if a patient is in a coma, unconscious, mentally challenged and so on), the physician must always assume that the patient is capable of making autonomous decisions. Anything less, may result in erroneously undermining innocent and healthy senses of patient autonomy, and this is not productive in ensuring effective communication between physician and patient.

Notes

1. By intrinsic tensions is meant personal character traits, or clashes in values or a lack of trust between the two parties; by extrinsic tensions is meant irrational dislikes or unwarranted condescension towards the patient.
2. By 'psychological competency' is meant intelligence and emotional perspicuity.
3. Steven Katz in his *The Silent World of Doctor and Patient* refers to this as the 'tension of authority'.

Chapter 7

Effective Communication

Effective communication is the building block for an effective physician-patient relationship which is complex due to the intrinsic vulnerabilities of medicine and the illness of the patient. In this chapter, I will focus on the essential features of effective communication to ensure that a patient achieves an informed consent. The thesis of this chapter is that effective communication is unachievable without honesty since it is the bedrock of all significant relationships. There are at least three features of effective communication that will ultimately result in an effective physician-patient relationship:

I.   Honesty;
II. Promise keeping/confidentiality; and
III. Caring and empathy.

These three conditions are the foundations for building effective communication and an effective physician-patient relationship. Honesty seems to be the overarching virtue in this triad since without it, the other two conditions cannot be achieved. For instance, if a physician and patient are honest with one another, there is a high probability that they will keep promises. Other times, owing to an empathetic attitude towards the patient, the physician will be honest with a patient. Being empathetic means that the physician would have to put him/herself in the patient's medical predicaments, and try to feel "what it would be like" to endure the patient's pain, distress and anxiety. Obviously, the physician can only form an imaginative analogue of the patient's health discomforts; however, this is sufficient to connect interpersonally with the patient. Being empathetic in this way will give the physician a proper appreciation of the patient's discomfort, and this, in turn, will enhance his/her ability to effectively communicate with one another.

The physician-patient relationship is unique since the two individuals usually enter into it involuntarily. The physician is usually regarded as a professional that can alleviate pain and suffering and/or give medical advice to a patient. At the beginning of the physician-patient relationship, there is an inequality between the two parties in that the patient is dependent on the physician for medical advice. If the relationship is to become effective, however, the texture of the relationship must change from a relationship of unequals to one of equals. This will ensure that the physician and patient will communicate openly and honestly with one another. The physician must recognize that his/her patient is a person whose bodily organs and functions are temporarily incapacitated by illness and in need of medical advice. However, the patient's sense of autonomy should not be undermined, although the patient's ability to make autonomous decisions may be weakened to some degree. The physician must always assume that the patient is capable of making autonomous decisions. Without effective communication, the patient would be unable to understand his/her treatment options in order to decide in favor of one of them. Thus, effective communication is an important condition for achieving an informed consent.

1.   Honesty[1]

Honesty is the first and most important condition for effective communication. The principle of honesty is a complex notion since it has a multitude of possible psychological, moral and religious connotations all of which may change the meaning of the term for each context in which the word is used. Generally, an individual is honest if s(he) is fair and sincere in both his/her personal character and behavior, and is not deceitful or untrustworthy. In this section, I will examine two kinds of honesty which are required for informed consent:

(1) Physician honesty; and
(2) Patient honesty.

(1) *Physician honesty.* In the medical context, physician honesty consists of: (1) an adequate description of the diagnosis and treatments available to the patient; (2) adequately disclosing the information in terms that can be understood by the patient; (3) being prudent not to bias a patient's response in favor of a certain treatment(s); and (4) avoiding intentionally deceiving a patient through exaggerations such as "if you don't undergo treatment X, you will surely die". These characteristics of honesty should be carefully considered by physicians to ensure that an honest exchange with the patient will result, and that an informed consent will be achieved.

It is not uncommon for physicians to engage in deliberate disingenuousness about a particular medical treatment without saying anything that is explicitly false to the patient.[2] The situation of deliberate deceit is not generally distinct from lying since if the physician intends to deceive, s(he) intended to lie, and therefore the physician's action will be morally wrong since deception of this kind undermines a patient's autonomy and right to make a decision that is based on a substantial disclosure of all the known treatments and their risks and benefits. The American Medical Association's "Principles of Ethics" of 1980 insists that the physician "deal honestly with patients and colleagues and strive to expose those physicians deficient in character or competence, or who engage in fraud and deception."[3]

There are two common types of dishonesty in the physician-patient relationship:

(i) Deception; and
(ii) Lying.

Sometimes deception is characterized in terms of lying. However, I argue that the two terms have distinct meanings, since although the terms aim at a similar result (being dishonest to a patient), their intention has different degrees and intensities. Lying is a much more direct form of dishonesty than deception which may be considered as being indirect. Furthermore, some physicians believe that deception is justified in some circumstances.

(i) *Deception.* A is deceived by B if B persuades A of something that is false or B misleads A into thinking something is the case when in fact it is not. Most cases of deception in the medical context is voluntary in nature. The act of deception has three elements: (a) evasion; (b) digression; and (c) distortion. I will examine each in turn.

(a) *Evasion* occurs when B diverts A's attention to another issue that is irrelevant to the main issue(s), so that A will believe differently as a result. Evasion also occurs when, for example, a patient's questions are not answered directly which may lead a patient to believe that his/her question was not important or by focusing on a similar question that doesn't address some of the patient's main concerns.

(b) *Digression* occurs when B intentionally focuses on another aspect of the medical situation instead of focusing on what A is strictly concerned with. This kind of response on the part of the physician is disrespectful of the patient as a person since it inadvertently gives the message that the patient's opinion is not worth the physician's consideration. In any effective physician-patient relationship, the patient's opinion is critically important, and it is not to be dismissed by ignoring it.

(c) *Distortion* of information occurs when B reinterprets the facts initially understood by A and expresses them in a way that is ambiguous or vague in relation to A's initial interpretation. Such a response ignores the patient's genuine medical concerns, and therefore disrespects his/her sense of self. Physician's must never, under any circumstances, *pretend* that their interpretation of the patient's medical situation is more accurate than the patient's own interpretation.

All of these forms of deception are morally wrong because they undermine a patient's autonomy and right to self-determination. On the autonomy-enhancing model, it can never be permissible to intentionally or unintentionally use any of the above forms of deception in any part of the process of communicating the medical treatments. If a physician is aware that the patient fails to understand some aspect of the medical treatment, this should be honestly communicated to the patient. Any form of deception undermines the fabric of the individual's character and erodes the possibility of an effective physician and patient relationship. Some forms of deception may indeed be unintentional since the physician may not intend to deceive a patient. However, once the physician becomes aware that s(he) has deceived the patient, an honest physician must disclose this fact to the patient. This will help to avoid any possible misunderstandings between physician and patient for future encounters.

(ii) *Lying* is distinguished from deception by being a direct utterance of a false statement. It occurs when messages are communicated to another individual with the explicit intention to mislead them and make them believe as true what the other individual believes is false. In short, to lie is to persuade someone to hold a false belief as if it were true. False statements are sometimes made to undermine a patient's interpretation of certain medical facts. A physician who lies to a patient is operating under the old traditional, paternalistic view of the physician-patient relationship where the physician may believe that lying to a patient is justified in order to get the patient to agree with a particular treatment. Such paternalism obviously undermines the patient's autonomy, and the consent that the patient gives for treatment can never be informed. To build an effective relationship that is based on effective communication, the physician must respect the patient's sense of personhood and autonomy. When a physician lies to a patient, s(he) destroys the possibility of effective communication and an effective physician-patient relationship.

In addition, when a physician intentionally lies to a patient, s(he) is undermining a patient's basic human right to decide for him/herself what treatment will be administered to his/her body to cure the patient's illness. Every patient has a right to a full disclosure of all the treatments, including all the risks and benefits. A physician that intentionally withholds such information does not respect the autonomy of the patient, and stifles any possibility of experiencing open, honest, communication that leads to mutual trust and respect. Only such a closely knit relationship between physician and patient could survive all the vulnerabilities created by the medical situation in which illness, pain and suffering dominate the relation.

2. *Patient honesty.* The patient also has a duty to be honest with the physician since the relationship between physician and patient is based on a reciprocal relationship of mutual trust and respect. Most patients are not intentionally dishonest with their physicians since it is not in their best interest to do so. Due to the vulnerabilities of illness and disease, and the pain and suffering that accrues as a result, the patient may sometimes either exaggerate the symptoms or underestimate the pain and suffering that (s)he is enduring. This is the case when illness makes a patient overly anxious or get into a state of denial about his/her illness. Once a certain set of facts is communicated by the patient to the physician, the physician must respond on the basis of the patient's assessment of these facts. If this assessment is not accurate, the physician will have an inaccurate description of the patient's illness. This is problematic since the physician will be unable to make a precise diagnosis of the disease. The physician must recognize this psychological fact as a possibility for some patients to ensure the patient is not over or under-estimating his/her medical condition. This procedure is also beneficial to the patient since s(he) is given a reality check about his/her illness. In this way, the patient is usually able to step back from his/her medical symptoms and decide for him/herself whether his/her initial assessment was accurate.

Effective communication is impossible without honesty between physician and patient since honesty is a necessary condition for meaningful exchanges between the two individuals. Neither can mutual trust be fostered without honest, open communication. The purpose of communication is severely undermined when one person intentionally engages in deception; to communicate means, in principle, to convey true not false or misleading information to evoke understanding, and to transmit genuine feelings and emotions to an individual. A presupposition of such an exchange is that it be honest and forthright. There is no point in disclosing false information to another person since it is assumed that the information disclosed will be true unless the individual proves to be untrustworthy.

II. Promise Keeping/Confidentiality

Secondly, effective communication is also based on keeping personal information confidential. If the patient cannot assume that the physician will keep information about the patient's health condition confidential, the patient may be hindered from disclosing certain information to the physician, and open, honest communication will be stifled. Thus, promise-keeping is an important aspect of developing a physician-patient relationship that is based on mutual trust and respect. There are two kinds of promise keeping that is especially relevant in the medical setting:

(1) Patient confidentiality; and
(2) Physician confidentiality.

(1) *Physician Confidentiality.* When a patient discloses personal information about his/her health, s(he) implicitly expects that the physician will not break his/her implicit promise to keep the information confidential. The physician has a duty not to disclose personal information about a particular patient to relatives, friends, or colleagues without the patient's express permission.[5] When a physician breaches the patient's trust in this way, the relationship may be either partly damaged or completely ruined, depending on the kind of information that was disclosed. For some patients, even a one time breach of trust will put the relationship in jeopardy since the implicit trust in the relationship was severely undermined by not keeping certain information confidential.

The most important breach of physician confidentiality occurs when relatives insist that they be given certain important personal information about the patient because they feel that they have a right to know without the patient's consent. Some physicians would argue that this should not be considered a breach of confidentiality since it is disclosed to close relatives and not to strangers. I insist that any personal information disclosed about a patient to any third party (close relatives or complete strangers) without the express permission of the patient is considered to be an instance of a breach of trust. The physician's primary responsibility is to the patient and not to his/her relatives. The mere communication between the physician and a third party (i.e., a relative) without a patient's consent or presence is dishonest, and breaks the trust between the two individuals. Consider the following case:

> Nancy White, a 57 year old mother of two was admitted to the hospital to rule out breast cancer. Despite Nancy's apparent pain, she appeared to be a well-balanced and rational individual. This was especially apparent when the physician diagnosed her health condition, and the possibility of cancer. Nancy was reflective about the whole testing procedure and wanted to know whether she had cancer so that, if she did, she could take the necessary steps to stop the spread of the cancer. While the tests are being processed, Nancy's husband and daughters approach the physician and ask him to disclose the results of the tests to them prior to telling Nancy. The relatives tell the physician that Nancy is unable to handle bad news due to her fear of cancer. They further say that Nancy has been mentally distressed since she began having difficulties with her health and would appreciate it if the physician would disclose the test results to them prior to Nancy. The tests come back positive. What should the physician do?

It is obvious that Nancy has manipulative relatives. Nancy showed no sign of mental distress when the physician spoke to her. In fact, she exhibited no fears whatsoever, making it seem that these fears were projections that originated from Nancy's family. In spite of this fact, the physician has no implicit or explicit duty to disclose any such information to the relatives without the patient's express permission. The physician must therefore disclose the test results to Nancy first, and tell her about her relatives concern for knowing whether she had cancer. If Nancy then asked the physician to tell her relatives, then the physician would be required to do so. Otherwise, it is Nancy's prerogative whether or not she tells her relatives and when (and if) she decides to do so, but it is not the physician's.

Another way of ensuring that the physician remains honest with his/her patient, is for all third parties to speak to the physician in the presence of the patient in regard to his/her health. This helps to build patient trust in the physician and ensures that the patient will decide how much personal information to disclose to relatives. The physician should never decide how much information to disclose on his/her own. In the patient's absence, the physician should not disclose any personal information about a patient to relatives. Any such breach of confidentiality is not permissible if effective communication is to result between physician and patient.

There is an implicit moral relationship between the physician and patient, and the confidentiality issue highlights this relation sharply. The physician must act on the principle of fidelity with regard to his/her patient, by consistently being loyal to the patient. This aspect of the physician-patient relationship may seem controversial since one may ask "Why does the physician have a duty to be morally bound to the patient?" The answer is quite obvious: Fidelity to a patient's concerns is necessary since a trusting patient-physician relationship cannot be built without securing a patient's confidential information. In addition, effective communication is enhanced if a physician is loyal to the patient.

(2) *Patient Confidentiality*. The physician must also trust that the patient will keep certain medical information confidential. These may be facts about the uncertainties of certain treatments or some experimental methods of treatment. In an effective physician-patient relationship, the physician may disclose information about gaps in his/her medical knowledge, fears that the outcome of certain treatments are more risky than others, confidence about administering certain

treatments over others, and so on. The physician expects that the patient will keep such information confidential. Thus, the physician and patient are morally bound to one another in a manner that should keep all third parties extrinsic to the relationship. This is the only way of ensuring that an effective physician-patient relationship will be secure, amidst the typical vulnerabilities of the medical situation, and the problem of close relatives infringing on the patient's and physician's personal boundaries.

III. Caring and Empathy

Thirdly, effective communication is based on fostering an empathetic relationship between physician and patient. One important feature of empathy is being in "communion" or "synchrony" with another individual. The empathizer (i.e., the physician) can initially better understand what the patient is experiencing by his/her verbal reports and body language. The physician can apprehend the patient's medical situation if: (i) s(he) has already experienced the medical condition first-hand; (2) if s(he) has seen someone close to him/her (a family member or friend) experience a similar medical situation second-hand; and (3) if s(he) can form a mental representation or analogue of the situation. One or more of the three conditions are necessary if the physician is to effectively empathize with the patient, since empathy is imaginatively reflecting on "what it would be like" to be in the patient's medical situation.

If a physician genuinely cares for his/her patient, s(he) will be empathetic with his/her pain, suffering and vulnerabilities. By being empathetic, the physician will be able to put himself/herself in the patient's shoes, and ask "What would it be like for me to have the illness my patient is enduring". In this way, the physician will be able to better understand the patient's predicament and will be able to communicate more effectively with his/her patient. Without an empathetic attitude by the physician towards the patient, the physician-patient relationship remains strictly professional, which hinders the active/interactive response that is necessary to communicate honestly and effectively. The patient must feel comfortable and at ease with his/her physician in order to ask further questions about the treatments without the physician being judgmental.

One theme of the book has been that the physician must understand the patient interpersonally by being cognizant of the patient's values, goals, beliefs, long and short term goals, intellectual capacity, and personal character traits in order for him/her to clearly communicate the medical treatments to the patient, and to ensure that the patient will make an autonomous decision in favor of a medical treatment. Such an appreciation of the patient's personal self is only possible through an empathetic, caring and responsible relationship with the patient, one that will allow the patient's personal idiosyncrasies to emerge. The patient must feel that the physician is treating him/her as a unique and special person and not only a diseased body. To treat the whole person, the physician must recognize the patient's personal idiosyncrasies and accept them uncritically, and to be acutely aware of the way illness and disease causes inherent vulnerabilities in all human beings. These vulnerabilities could be lessened by the physician through an empathetic interaction with the patient, which presupposes that the physician is non-judgmental, open, kind, honest and harmonious with the patient. This further presupposes that the physician must be an altruistic and compassionate person, one who feels intrinsically connected to his/her patients. This connection is sometimes referred to as "fellow feeling" which is a feeling of good will towards all human beings. The physician must feel that s(he) can be of assistance to his/her patient in a way that transcends medical boundaries and reaches the patient in his/her own personal idiosyncrasies as a unique individual.

An empathetic attitude towards a patient also facilitates recovery from an illness. The empathetic physician is able to positively encourage a patient by empowering the patient to take the necessary small steps on the path to recovery from surgery or other painful treatments. Patients usually need to realize that they do matter to the physician, and that s(he) really cares about the patient's well-being. The patient must feel that the physician genuinely wants the patient to progressively get healthier until his/her medical condition is alleviated and the patient is healthy again. Such a positive and encouraging attitude is crucial for quick recovery.

Honesty is the bedrock of all medical interactions in the medical setting and of establishing effective communication between physician and patient that will yield an informed consent. A substantial disclosure of the medical treatments for a given illness, understanding these treatments and making a rational, reflective and well informed decision in favor of a treatment are all impossible to achieve without an effective physician-patient relationship that stresses honest, empathetic interactions. The texture of the physician-patient relationship must change from the old traditional paradigm of the professional, paternalistic physician to an empathetic, honest and trustworthy physician. To be more precise, the physician-patient relationship must be changed from a relationship of unequals (on the paternalistic model) to a relationship of equals (on the autonomy-enhancing model). The physician and patient relationship must be regarded as an equal partnership that is formed for the purpose of alleviating a patient's unique and idiosyncratic health problems.

Notes

1. Honesty in medical contexts is an important problem. The following articles are only a sample of the debate currently in progress:

> Jackson, Jennifer. "Telling The Truth". *Journal of Medical Ethics*, 17 (1991), 5-9.
>
> Minogue, Brendan, P., & Taraszewski. "The Whole Truth and Nothing But The Truth?" *Hastings Center Report*, (October-November, 1988), 34-36.
>
> Novack, Dennis, H., Deterring, Barbara, J., Arnold, Robert, Forrow, Lachlan, Landinsky, Morissa, & Pezullo, John, C. "Physicians' Attitudes Toward Using Deception to Resolve Difficult Ethical Problems". *Journal of American Medical Association*, 261(20), (1989), 2980-2985.

2. Michael Lockwood. *Moral Dilemmas in Modern Medicine*, chapter on "The Truth" by Roger Higgs, p. 187-202.

3. Lockwood, p. 190.

4. In this section, I will first focus primarily on the physician's responsibility to keep information confidential since it seems that there is a greater tendency for the physician to disclose confidential information to third parties than for the patient to do so.

5. The only condition under which physicians could disclose information about the patient to the nursing staff or any other medical practitioners is if such individuals are directly responsible for the medical treatment of the patient. Even in those cases, the patient should be explicitly aware who the information is disclosed to. However, no information about the patient should be disclosed to any other individuals without the patient's express permission.

Chapter 8

Paradigm Shift in Informed Consent

Informed consent is presently at the crossroads between the traditional, paternalistic, harm-avoidance model and the autonomy-enhancing, patient-oriented model. I will analyze the two models and assess each in terms of their moral and medical efficacy. The autonomy-enhancing, patient-oriented model focuses on the process of giving an informed consent in favor of a medical treatment that has been autonomously decided by the patient. The harm avoidance-model stresses the paternalistic, authoritative physician-centered model in which the patient consents to treatment by passively and non-autonomously accepting the treatment prescribed by the physician. This is precisely what the autonomy-enhancing model rejects since a patient cannot give an informed consent without making an autonomous decision in favor of a medical treatment. On the paternalistic model, the only purpose of consent is for the patient to agree with the physician's suggested treatment.

It then follows that on the traditional/paternalistic model, the consent required cannot be informed since it is merely a legal formality in which the patient's signature is required on a form. The ultimate purpose of consent, on this model, is to reduce any possible legal culpability by the medical staff should any health complications arise. However, this undermines the genuine purpose of informed consent which is to honor a patient's right to self-determination and autonomy. On the traditional/paternalistic paradigm, a patient's agreement with a particular medical treatment (chosen by the physician) is all there is to which consent is needed. In other words, as long as the patient is aware of the most probable risks that are possible for one of the treatments available, s(he) has given consent. The kind of consent that is required by a physician on the traditional model cannot be considered 'informed'; instead, it is merely an 'agreement' by a patient to allow a certain treatment. However, an agreement does not constitute an   informed consent, since informed consent is much more than an agreement. It is an autonomous decision that is achieved by understanding all the treatments disclosed by the physician and making a rational decision in favor of a treatment, and not merely that which the physician considers to be the most appropriate. Thus, the traditional view of informed consent is negligent in determining what precisely constitutes an informed consent, since the physician fails to disclose all of the medical treatments to the patient. The result is that it is inconceivable on the traditional model for the patient to make an autonomous decision in favor of a medical treatment that is based on a substantial disclosure since the treatment is chosen by the physician without consulting the patient.

Thus, on the traditional paternalistic model, the physician decides which treatment is best for the patient, a decision which is based solely on his/her medical expertise and has very little, if anything, to do with the patient as a person (his/her values, goals, life plans, beliefs and so on). This view of informed consent is inadequate since it avoids the ultimate purpose of an informed consent, which is to allow the patient to achieve an autonomous, reflective decision in favor of a medical treatment that is in harmony with the patient's values and beliefs. What the harm-avoidance model lacks then is any recognition that illness is a lived experience for some particular patient and this illness cannot be treated merely as an objective, medical phenomenon, in abstraction from the patient's experience. In other words, the patient should not merely be treated as a diseased body but rather as a person with a disease.

I. Subjective versus Objective Models of Informed Consent

When a patient is merely treated objectively by a physician (which is required by the harm-avoidance model), s(he) feels undermined as an autonomous person. There is no need for developing an adequate physician-patient relationship since the physician is regarded as a medical expert that a patient consults for medical advice. What is missing in this account is the effect that an illness has on a patient's life and psychological well-being. This is especially the case for chronic illness patients (such as chronic asthma or cancer patients) where the illness must become integrated into a patient's lifestyle and become part of the patient's self-experience. The patient's self or sense of personhood qualitatively changes with the occurrence of disease since pain and physical incapabilities become an integral part of the patient's everyday life. For cancer patients, for instance, the effects of radiation therapy or chemotherapy has a drastic effect on their physical and psychological well-being, a discomfort that never leaves the patient, not even when s(he) is asleep. Thus, when a physician treats the patient objectively, all their subjective, personal pains and discomforts are largely unrecognized and the patient may even feel more vulnerable and ill as a result.

The autonomy-enhancing view advocated throughout the book incorporates a subjective-objective model of informed consent. The subjective component includes the patient's values, beliefs and goals, and is just as significant as the objective component which includes the patient's medical history and present medical condition. The five conditions on the autonomy-enhancing model I have outlined in the previous chapters includes both the subjective and objective components of an informed consent, although the major focus has been on the subjective. I have assumed that the main difficulty of achieving informed consent does not rest so much on a physician's medical expertise, diagnosis of illness, or even on the possible gaps in his/her medical knowledge, as on the importance of including the patient into the choosing of the treatment options available to the patient. On the

autonomy-enhancing model, the personal/ subjective features are central
to the process of deriving an informed consent. When the Hippocratic
Oath was developed in the fourth century B.C. and established as a code
of Ethics for medical professionals, paternalism was the only accepted
view among medical practitioners. At the time, this oath was an
important advancement in medical practice, and it continued to be well
into the twentieth century. However, after the second world war, views
fundamentally changed with regard to informed consent for a number of
possible reasons.[1]   First, the emerging legal doctrine brought the
concept of "Informed Consent" to the attention of the medical
community. Shortly thereafter, "informed consent" was extended to
form a new medical ethics focusing on decisional authority and the
physician-patient relationship. The debate is still very much underway
and it is perhaps for this reason that most physicians still fluctuate
between the traditional model and the autonomy-enhancing model.
Secondly, the law and ethics were influenced by the increasingly
technological, powerful and impersonal medical care at a time when
individuals in society became preoccupied with liberty, autonomy and
social equality. Individuals insisted to be part of the process of making
the important medical decisions in their lives. Thirdly, there were the
Nazi atrocities and the well-known cases of abuse on research subjects
in the U.S. which raised suspicions as to the trustworthiness of the
medical profession. The "Patient's Bill of Rights" of 1972 was passed
to insist on better medical care as well as to change the paradigm of
patient respect.

II. The Shift to Informed Consent

The paradigm of informed consent began to change from a
physician-oriented process that was based on the harm avoidance model
and the Hippocratic Oath, to a much more patient-oriented process in
the early 1970s at a time when we became an autonomy-oriented
culture. The Hippocratic Oath was developed due to a public concern for
physician responsibility towards patients. It focuses on the professional
conduct of physicians' paternalistic medical care. The oath fails to
address some of the key issues of informed consent such as: disclosure,

understanding of the treatment options, communication, respecting a patient's decisions, and an open and caring physician-patient relationship, all of which are necessary conditions for achieving an 'informed' consent. Instead, it focuses on an unreflective type of paternalism advising physicians to

> conceal most things from the patient, while you are attending to him ... turning his attention away from what is being done to him; ... revealing nothing of the patient's future or present condition.[2]

The physician is portrayed as someone who commands and decides, while patients must comply with a physician's decisions. This kind of paternalistic care may still be prevalent in some medical societies.

For a reciprocal physician-patient relationship, the oath must be reformulated and reinterpreted. The purpose of medicine must be extended to include a cordial and caring attitude towards patients that transcends medical boundaries. The change in view presupposes that physician and patient must enter into a partnership-type relationship in which both are equal partners. The previously presupposed power imbalance must be altered if patients are to achieve informed consent. In fact, an informed consent, given its inherent complexities, cannot be achieved in any other way. Physicians and patients are both knowledgeable and have something essential to contribute to the process of informed consent. The physician has medical expertise to cure the patient's illness, and the patient has self-knowledge to contribute to the process of informed consent. Both kinds of expertise are essential to achieving an informed consent.

The paradigm shift in medicine from the harm avoidance model to the autonomy-enhancing model has still not been completely accomplished. However, progress is being made and medical schools in Canada now encourage physicians to develop important personal attitudes in which their interactions with patients is much more personal, and a patient is encouraged to make an autonomous, rational decision in favor of a medical treatment.[3] Some physicians who are still partial to the traditional, paternalistic paradigm often swing back and forth from the autonomy-enhancing model to the harm-avoidance model, depending on the patient or medical situation.[4] This is especially the case for general practitioners who tend to service many patients, with less time for individual patients, and discovering who they are as persons. Specialists usually give much more personal attention to patients; however, only some specialists adopt the autonomy-enhancing model which requires that they get to know the patient's values and goals. Physicians, in general, still feel more comfortable with the harm-avoidance model of patient care, with the inclusion of a few features from the autonomy-enhancing model since they still view medicine as an objective enterprise with very few subjective elements. Some physicians believe that bringing in subjective elements will make the process of giving an informed consent far too difficult to achieve, and it gives physicians extra burdens that extend far beyond their call of duty, which is chiefly to restore health and cure illness. One of the main themes of this book has been that an informed consent is impossible to achieve by strict adherence to the harm-avoidance model, and that unless the physician takes some (if not all) of the patient's personal features into account, the whole purpose of informed consent which is to honor a patient's autonomy, is undermined. Bringing the patient as a person into the process of informed consent may be more difficult due to the idiosyncrasies of each individual patient; however, the patience and effort that are required to achieve this is well worth the effort that it takes.

The autonomy-enhancing model outlined in this book ensures that the patient enters into a partnership with the physician and becomes actively involved in the process of achieving an autonomous, reflective and rational decision in favor of a medical treatment. The primary focus is on the patient, and the process involved in giving an informed consent is a result of active, personal interaction with the physician. If a patient makes a decision in favor of a treatment that is not autonomous, s(he) has not given an informed consent. The most important aspect of an informed consent is that the patient makes a substantially autonomous decision in favor of a medical treatment, which consists of: (1) assessing the patient's sense of autonomy and mental competency (which are two foundational elements necessary for an informed consent), and (2) adhering to the suggested five stage conditional process.[5] This constitutes a new paradigm for informed consent, one that can ensure that a patient achieves an informed consent.

Thus, an effective physician patient relationship that is based on mutual trust, respect, honesty and caring is impossible to achieve on the traditional, paternalistic model. A new model is necessary for achieving informed consent that is based on an autonomous, reflective, rational, substantially understood medical treatments that is substantially disclosed to the patient. The autonomy-enhancing model may be considered as a new ideology for achieving an informed consent. Thus, a paradigm shift from the traditional, harm-avoidance model to the autonomy-enhancing model is absolutely necessary to ensure that physicians get an "informed" consent for medical treatments, but not mere 'consent', which is unreflective, non-autonomous and uninformed. Physicians should accept the challenges of changing the paradigm of informed consent from the harm-avoidance model to the autonomy-enhancing model. Only in this way can a truly informed consent be achieved.

Notes

1. The impetus for this discussion about the reasons for the changed views on informed consent are derived from Ruth Faden and Tom Beauchamp's *A History and Theory of Informed Consent* (New York: Oxford University Press, 1986), p. 86-89.
2. This quote is from the selections from the Hippocratic Corpus, Decorum, XVI, in W.H.S. Jones, *Hippocrates* (4 volumes) (Cambridge, Mass.: Harvard University Press, 1923-31, 2:297, 229).
3. One such medical school is The McMaster Medical School in Ontario, Canada, which is focusing on developing certain character traits in physicians in responding to their patients on a personal level.
4. If a patient has a reflective disposition, the physician may advocate the autonomy-enhancing model of informed consent, whereas if a patient is

unreflective, the physician will simply suggest a treatment on the patient's behalf.

5.   The Foundational elements are analyzed and assessed in Chapter 1 and 2, whereas the conditional elements are analyzed in chapters 3-7.

Bibliography

Alfidi, Ralph, J. "Informed Consent: A Study of Patient Reaction".
The Journal of American Medical Association. Volume 216(8),
1971, 1325-1329.

Annas, George, J. "Whose Waste Is It Anyway? The Case of John
Moore". *Hastings Center Report,* (October-November, 1988),
37-39.

Applebaum, Paul, S., Lidz, Charles, W., & Meisel, Alan. *Informed
Consent: Legal Theory and Clinical Practice.* New York: Oxford
University Press, 1987.

Beasley, Alfred, D., & Graber, Glenn, C. "The Range of Autonomy:
Informed Consent in Medicine". *Theoretical Medicine,* 5 (1984)
31-41.

Beauchamp, T., & Childress, J. *Principles of Biomedical Ethics.* New
York: Oxford University Press, 1979.

Beauchamp, T., & McCullough, L. *Medical Ethics: The
Responsibility of Physicians.* Englewoods Cliffs: Prentice Hall,
Inc., 1984.

Bennett, Henry, L. "Trees and Heads: The Objective and the
Subjective in Painful Procedures". *The Journal of Clinical Ethics,*
5(3), (1994), 149-151.

Brody, H. "Transparency: Informed Consent in Primary Care".
Hastings Centre Report. Volume 19, 1989, 5-9.

Buchanan, Allen, B. *Deciding for Others: The Ethics of Surrogate
Decision Making.* New York: Cambridge University Press, 1992.

Buehler, David, A. "Informed Consent - Wishful Thinking?" *Journal
of Medical and Human Bioethics.* Volume 4, 1982, 43-57.

Bulmer, Martin. *Social Research Ethics.* New York: Holmes and
Meier, 1982.

Campbell, Alastair, V. *Moderated Love: A Theology of Professional Care*. London: SPCK Book Publishers, 1984.

Carr, Craig, L. "Tacit Consent". *Public Affairs Quarterly*, 4(4), 1990, 335-344.

Cassell, Eric, J. "The Function of Medicine". *Hastings Center Report*, (1977), 16-19.

Clouser, Danner, K., & Gert, Bernard. "A Critique of Principalism". *The Journal of Medicine and Philosophy*, 15 (1990), 219-236.

Coleman, Lester, L. "The Patient-Physician Relationship". *Physician's World*, 1974.

Dagi, Forcht, Teo. "Changing the Paradigm for Informed Consent". *The Journal of Clinical Ethics*, 5(3) (1994), 246-250.

Drane, James, F. *Becoming a Good Doctor: The Place of Virtue and Character in Medical Ethics*. Kansas, MO: Sheed & Ward, 1988.

Drane, James, F. "The Many Faces of Competency". *Hastings Centre Report*. Volume 15, 1985, 17-21.

Dunstan, G.R., and Seller, Mary J. *Consent in Medicine: Convergence and Divergence in Tradition*. England: Hallen Street Press, 1983.

Dworkin, Gerald. *The Theory and Practice of Autonomy*. Cambridge: Cambridge University Press, 1988.

Elias, Sherman, & Annas, George, J. "The Whole Truth and Nothing But the Truth?" *Hastings Centre Report*, Volume 18, 1988, 35-36.

Emanuel, Ezekiel, J. & Emanuel, Linda, L. "Four Models of the Physician-Patient Relationship". *Journal of American Medical Association*, 267(16), (1992), 2221-2226.

Faden, Ruth, R., & Beauchamp, Tom L. *A History and Theory of Informed Consent*. New York: Oxford University Press, 1986.

Fromer, Margot, Joan. *Ethical Issues in Health Care*. St. Louis: Mosby, 1981.

Garrett, Thomas, M., & Baille, Harold, W. *Health Care Ethics*. Englewood Cliffs: Prentice Hall, 1989.

Gillon, Raanan. *Principles of Health Care Ethics*. New York: John Willey & Sons, 1994.

Gillon, Raanan. "Medical Ethics in Britain". *Theoretical Medicine*, Volume 9, 1988, 251-269.

Gillon, Raanan. *Philosophical Medical Ethics*. New York: John Wiley & Sons, 1985.

Gorovitz, Samule, Macklin, Ruth, Jameton, Andrew, L., O'Connor, J., and Sherwin, Susan. *Moral Problems in Medicine.* New Jersey: Prentice Hall, 1983.

Graber, Glenn, C., Beasley, Alfred D., and Eaddy, John A. *Ethical Analysis of Clinical Medicine: A Guide to Self-Evaluation.* Baltimore, Munich: Urban and Schwarzenberg, 1985.

Gunderson, Martin. "Justifying a Principle of Informed Consent: A Case Study in Autonomy-Based Ethics." *Public Affairs Quarterly,* Volume 4(3), 249-265, 1990.

Hull, Richard, T. "Informed Consent: Patient's Right or Patient's Duty." *Journal of Medical Philosophy.* Volume 10, 1985, 183-198.

Inman, W.H.W. "Risks in Medical Intervention: Balancing Therapeutic Risks and Benefits", in *The Future of Predictive Safety Evaluation.* Lancaster: MTP Press, Limited, 1986.

Jackson, Jennifer. "Telling The Truth". *Journal of Medical Ethics,* 17 (1991), 5-9.

Jacobson, Jay, A. "Informed Consent: Pondering a New Piece of the Puzzle". *The Journal of Clinical Ethics,* 5(3), (1994), 244-246.

Kahneman, Daniel, & Tversky, Amos. "Choices, Frames and Values". *American Psychologist,* 1984, Volume 39(4), 341-350.

Kantor, Jay, E. *Medical Ethics for Physicians-in-Training.* New York: Plenum Medical Book Company, 1989.

Katz, Jay. *The Silent World of Doctor and Patient.* New York: Free Press, 1984.

Kelly, Michael, J. "Should Competence be Coerced?" *Hastings Centre Report,* 1990, Volume 20(4), 31-32.

Lammers, Stephen, E., & Verhey, Allen. *On Moral Medicine.* Michigan: William B. Erdmans Publishing Company.

Lockwood, Michael. *Moral Dilemmas in Modern Medicine.* Oxford: Oxford University Press, 1985.

MacNiven, Donald. "Patients' Rights and The Doctor-Patient Relationship". *Renaissance Universal Journal,* 1984, Volume 4, 2-3.

Marcus, Ruth, B. "Uninformed Consent". *Science.* 1979, 644-647.

McCullough, Laurence, & Christianson, Charles. "Ethical Dimensions of Diagnosis". *Metamedicine,* 1981, Vol. 2, 129-141.

Miller, Bruce, L. "Autonomy and the Refusal of Lifesaving Treatment". *The Hastings Center Report,* (1981), 22-28.

Minogue, Brendan, P., & Taraszewski. "The Whole Truth and Nothing But The Truth?" *Hastings Center Report,* (October-November, 1988), 34-36.

Morreim, Haavi. "Three Concepts of Patient Competence". *Theoretical Medicine,* 4 (1983), 231-252.

Novack, Dennis, H., Detering, Barbara, J., Arnold, Robert, Forrow, Lachlan, Landinsky, Morissa, & Pezullo, John, C. "Physicians' Attitudes Toward Using Deception to Resolve Difficult Ethical Problems". *Journal of American Medical Association,* 261(20), (1989), 2980-2985.

O'Rourke, Kevin, & Brodeur, Dennis. *Medical Ethics: Common Ground For Understanding.* St. Louis: The Catholic Health Association of the United States, 1986.

Parsons, T. "The Sick role and the Role of the Physician Reconsidered". *Milbank Memorial Fund Quarterly,* 1975, 257-275.

Patients' Rights in Ontario. Toronto: Patients' Rights Association, 1982.

Perry, Clifton, "Negligence in Securing Informed Consent and Medical Malpractice". *Journal of Medical and Human Bioethics.* 1988, Volume 9, 111-120.

Reamer, Frederic, G. "Should Competence be Coerced?"*Hastings Centre Report,* 1990, 30-32.

Rosenberg, James, A., & Towers, Bernard. "The Practice of Empathy as a Prerequisite for Informed Consent". *Theoretical Medicine,* 1986, Volume 7, 181-194.

Robbins, Dennis, A. *Ethical Dimensions of Clinical Medicine.* Springfield: Thomas, 1981.

Rosenberg, James, E., & Toweres, Bernard. "The Practice of Empathy as a Prerequisite for Informed Consent". *Theoretical Medicine,* 7 (1986), 181-194.

Self, Donnie. "The Pedagogy of Two Different Approaches to Humanistic Medical Education: Cognitive vs. Affective". *Theoretical Medicine*, 9 (1988), 227-236.

Slovic, Paul. "Perception of Risk". *Science*, 236 (1987), 280-285.

Smith, David, H. *Respect and Care in Medical Ethics*. Lanham: University Press of America, 1985.

Somerville, Margaret, A. *Consent to Medical Care*. A Study Paper Prepared for the Law Reform Commission of Canada.

Spicker, Stuart, F., & Ratzan, Richard, M. "*ARS MEDICINA ET CONDITIO HUMANA*: Edmund D. Pellegrino, M.D., on His 70th Birthday". *The Journal of Medicine and Philosophy*, 15 (1990), 327-341.

Sulmasy, Daniel, P., Lehmann, Lisa, S., Levine, David, M., & Faden, Ruth. "Patients' Perceptions of the Quality of Informed Consent for Common Medical Procedures". *The Journal of Clinical Ethics*, 5(3), (1994), 189-195.

Thomas, John, E. *Medical Ethics and Human Life*. Toronto: Samuel Stevens, 1983.

Thomas, John, E., & Waluchow, Wilfred. *Well and Good: Case Studies in Biomedical Ethics*. Ontario: Broadview Press, Ltd., 1987.

Thomasma, David, C. "Establishing the Moral Basis of Medicine: Edmund D. Pellegrino's Philosophy of Medicine". *The Journal of Medicine and Philosophy*, 15 (1990), 245-267.

Turner, Gerald, P., & Mapa, Joseph. *Humanistic Health Care: Issues for Caregivers*. Ann Arbor, Michigan: Health Administration Press, 1988.

Tversky, Amos. "Elimination by Aspects". *Pyschological Review*. Volume 79(4), 1972, 281-299.

Tversky, Amos, & Kahneman, Daniel. "The Framing of Decisions and the Psychology of Choice". *Science*, Volume 211, 453-458, 1981.

Tversky, Amos, & Kahneman, Daniel. "Judgment Under Uncertainty". *Science*, Volume 85, 1124-1131, 1974.

Van De Veer, Donald. *Paternalistic Intervention: The Moral Bounds of Benevolence.* New Jersey: Princeton University Press, 1986.

Van De Veer, Donald. *Health Care Ethics.* Philadelphia: Temple University Press, 1982.

Veatch, Robert, M. "Abandoning Informed Consent". *Hastings Center Report,* (March-April, 1995), 5-12.

Veatch, Robert, M. *A Theory of Medical Ethics.* New York: Basic Books, Inc., 1981.

Veatch, Robert, M. "Why Get Consent?" *Hospital Physician.* Volume 11, 30-31, 1975.

Veatch, Robert, M. "Generalization of Expertise". *Hastings Centre Studies.* Volume 1(2), 29-40, 1973.

Vollrath, John. "Experiments and Rights". *Bioethics,* Volume 3, 93-105, 1989.

Warner, Richard. *Morality in Medicine.* Sherman Oaks: Alfred, 1980.

Wear, Stephen. "Patient Autonomy, Paternalism and the Conscientious Physician". *Theoretical Medicine,* 4, (1983), 253-274.

Wright, Richard, A. *Human Values in Health Care: The Practice of Ethics.* New York: McGraw Hill, 1988.

Young, Peter. *Personal Autonomy: Beyond Negative and Positive Liberty.* London: Croom Helm, 1986.

INDEX